Nursing Care Planning Guides

for

Psychiatric and Mental Health Care

Margo Creighton Neal, RN, MN*
President, Nurseco, Inc.

Patricia Feltz Cohen, RN, MN, EdM
Consultant
Huntington Beach, CA

Phyllis Gorney Cooper, RN, MN
Consultant
Los Angeles, CA

Joan Reighley, RN, MN**
Psychotherapist, private practice
Los Angeles, CA

*Certified, generalist; Division of Psychiatric and Mental Health Nursing, American Nurses' Association
**Certified, specialist; Division of Psychiatric and Mental Health Nursing, American Nurses' Association

Nurseco, Inc., Pacific Palisades, CA

© Copyright by Margo Creighton Neal, 1981. All rights reserved. No part of this book may be reproduced in any form or by any electronic or mechanical means, including information storage and retrieval systems, without permission in writing from the publisher except by a reviewer who may quote brief passages in a review.

Printed in the United States of America.

Published by NURSECO, Inc., 1011 Swarthmore, PO Box 145, Pacific Palisades, CA 90272.

First Printing, 1981.

Library of Congress Cataloging in Publication Data
Main entry under title:

Nursing care planning guides for psychiatric and mental health care.

    Includes index.
    1.   Psychiatric nursing. I. Neal, Margo Creighton, 1935- . [DNLM: 1. Patient care planning—Handbooks. 2. Psychiatric nursing—Handbooks. 3. Mental health services—Handbooks. WY 160 N9745]
RC440.N86   610.73'68   81-16824
ISBN 0-935236-15-5   AACR2

PREFACE

The nursing care of psychiatric and mental health patients is highly specialized. Consequently, we have brought together this edition of *Nursing Care Planning Guides for Psychiatric and Mental Health Care,* extrapolated from our five current sets of *Nursing Care Planning Guides.*

These Guides will give nurses some specific guidelines, suggestions, and recommendations to provide this specialized nursing care. They will also assist nurses in writing specific, individualized nursing care plans.

In some of the Guides we have attempted to avoid stereotyping the nurse as "she" and the patient as "he" by using "s/he" in lieu of she/he. However, since the English language has yet to produce a combination form for masculine and feminine pronouns, you will note some reference to the patient as masculine only.

The individual Guide numbers (e.g. NCP Guide No. 1:31) refer to the placement of the Guide in the originally published Sets. The number following is the page number of this edition.

Margo C. Neal
Patricia F. Cohen
Phyllis G. Cooper
Joan Reighley

FOREWORD

Each of the Nursing Care Planning Guides in this edition is written in the format of a nursing care plan. Each contains all the basic components: long-term goal, patient outcomes, areas of patient problems, and nursing actions.

In addition, each Guide contains a definition and "General Considerations," which provide a precis of background information specific to the condition. At the end of each Guide can be found possible discharge criteria and recommended readings.

To use these Guides most efficiently, scan the Table of Contents, then choose the ones specific to your patients, for example, "The Patient with Schizophrenia." The "General Considerations" component will help you do a patient assessment; the "Specific Considerations" will help you define the patient's individual needs, set short-term outcomes, and choose nursing interventions. You may also want to refer to those guides in the "Supplementary Information" section, e.g. "Drugs: Psychotropic."

These Nursing Care Planning Guides present guidelines, suggestions, recommendations; they are *not* standard nursing care plans. Nurses should take from them those aspects that can be applied to a specific patient, individualizing them as needed, and adding to them as they see fit.

In the settings of psychiatric and mental health nursing care, these Nursing Care Planning Guides can help you provide the highly specialized nursing care that is required.

Psychiatric and Mental Health Care
TABLE OF CONTENTS

A — The Adult Patient/Client

(1:20)	The Patient Manifesting Aggression	1
(2:01)	The Patient with Alcoholism	3
(1:21)	The Patient Manifesting Anger	7
(4:36)	The Patient with an Antisocial Personality	9
(1:22)	The Patient Experiencing Anxiety	11
(2:29)	The Patient Experiencing a Body Image Disturbance	13
(5:30)	The Patient Adapting to Chronic Illness Role	17
(1:23)	The Patient Experiencing Confusion	21
(2:31)	The Patient Needing Crisis Intervention	23
(1:24)	The Patient Manifesting Denial	27
(1:25)	The Patient Experiencing Dependency	29
(1:26)	The Patient Experiencing Depression	31
(3:35)	The Patient Experiencing Depression (Psychiatric)	33
(4:37)	The Patient with a Developmental Disability: Mental Retardation (in an Acute Setting)	39
(4:38)	The Client with a Developmental Disability: Mental Retardation (in a Residential Setting)	43
(1:28)	The Patient Experiencing Fear	49
(5:31)	The Patient Experiencing Guilt	51
(1:27)	Dealing with Impending Death	55
(5:32)	The Patient Experiencing a Threat to Self-Esteem	59
(3:36)	The Patient with Manic-Depressive Psychosis	63
(1:29)	The Patient Manifesting Manipulation	67
(5:33)	The Patient Manifesting Noncompliance	69
(1:30)	The Patient Experiencing Pain	73
(5:34)	The Patient Experiencing Powerlessness	77
(4:39)	The Victim of Rape/Sexual Assault	81
(3:37)	The Patient with Schizophrenia	87
(1:32)	The Patient Experiencing Sensory Disturbances	93
(5:35)	The Patient Experiencing Shame/Embarrassment	95
(1:33)	The Patient Experiencing Shock, Psychogenic	97
(5:36)	The Patient Adapting to the Sick Role	99
(3:38)	The Patient who is Suicidal (on a Psychiatric Unit)	103
(3:39)	The Patient who has Attempted Suicide (admitted to a Med-Surg. Unit)	107
(4:40)	The Patient who is Violent	111

B — The Child Patient/Client

(4:20)	The Child: Battered Child Syndrome	115
(4:25)	The Child who is Dying/Terminal	119
(4:21)	The Child with a Developmental Disability: Mental Retardation (in an Acute Setting)	123
(4:22)	The Child with a Developmental Disability: Mental Retardation (in a Residential Setting)	127
(4:27)	The Child Victim of Rape/Sexual Assault	131

C — Supplementary Information

(4:41)	Assessment of Mental Status	133
(5:37)	Behavior Modification	137
(2:35)	Crisis Intervention: Adaptation to General Nursing	141
(3:45)	Drugs: Hypnotics & Sedatives	145

(3:46)	Drugs: Psychotropic	147
(3:47)	Drugs: Tranquilizers (Minor)	151
(1:40)	Effects of Hospitalization: Part A: Tension-Producing Causes	153
(1:41)	Effects of Hospitalization: Part B: Assessment	155
(1:42)	Effects of Hospitalization: Part C: Prolonged Confinement	157
(4:46)	Evidence Collection: Rape/Sexual Assault	159
(3:24)	Normal Growth & Development: Toddler/Preschool	161
(3:25)	Normal Growth & Development: School Age Child	167
(3:26)	Normal Growth & Development: Adolescent	173
(2:49)	Problem-Oriented Charting	177
(5:47)	Problem-Solving	181
(1:31)	Responses to Loss: The Grief and Mourning Process	185
(1:48)	Steps in Writing Nursing Care Plans	187
(1:49)	Teaching Patients: General Suggestions	191
(1:50)	Teaching Patients: Specific Plan for Skills and Procedures	195

NCP Guide No. **1:20** 1

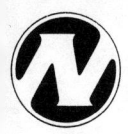

The Patient Manifesting Aggression

Definition: A forceful, attacking action, which may be physical, verbal or symbolic. It is unrealistic and directed toward the environment or inwardly toward the self.

LONG TERM GOAL: The patient will use realistic and self-protective (assertive) behavior to make known his needs and desires.

General Considerations:
— **Each aggressive incident should be reviewed** with a goal of improving patient care by identifying situations which contribute to aggression and by evaluating and revising interventions.
— **Nursing assessment** includes awareness of the behavioral manifestations of aggression which include:
  — overt, constant demands;
  — constant self-directed anger;
  — refusal to listen to staff;
  — constant or intermittent attempts at changing the plan of care;
  — abusive verbal language;
  — constant or intermittent non-adherence to Dr.'s orders.
— **Nursing responsibilities** include assessment of the patient's usual coping behaviors in order to recognize and support behaviors that are adaptive and positive.

Specific Considerations, Potential Patient Outcomes, and Nursing Actions:

1) Immediate Response to Recognition of Aggressive Behavior

The patient will limit or stop aggressive behavior:
— set limits on physically harmful behavior and explain to the pt. why you are doing so;
— contrast to the pt. his physical & emotional functioning that is realistic (assertive) versus that which is unrealistic and forceful (aggressive);
— always prepare the pt. (physically & verbally) for what you are going to do even if you consider it a daily and/or usual activity;
— encourage the pt. to express his feelings regarding the deprivation caused by the hospitalization & illness; sit down & listen; use open-ended questions;
— recognize that the pt.'s aggression may be in response to fear, increased dependency, &/or anxiety; therefore, do not attempt to defend yourself, the staff or the agency; listen to what the pt. is saying & assist him to understand his own method of coping.

2) Restoration to Adaptive Coping	The patient will utilize assertive behaviors as a means of expressing independence and control; will recognize and utilize outside sources of comfort and support:

- know the difference between assertive (asking for what one wants; standing up for rights) and aggressive behavior (getting what one wants *at the expense of others*);
- plan the nursing care & daily routine with the pt., giving him as much flexibility in decision-making as possible; evaluate the care with him;
- reinforce positive (assertive) approaches utilized by the pt. ("I would like . . ." versus "Do this . . .");
- give the pt. the opportunity to plan & do things s/he likes to do, i.e. sleeping late, knitting, reading;
- praise the pt.'s efforts to maintain independence & be assertive;
- explain the reason for the pt.'s behavior to his significant others (SO), i.e., it is his way of coping;
- praise the efforts of the SOs in their attempts to assist the pt. in coping;
- stress to staff the importance of not chastising or rejecting the pt. for his efforts to cope by using aggressive behavior; rather, set limits on behavior that is physically destructive & teach the patient to be assertive instead of aggressive.

Discharge Planning and Teaching Objectives/Outcomes
1) (Patient/Family/Significant Other) Can verbalize behavior or demands that trigger the protective response of aggression.
2) Can describe the difference between assertiveness and aggression.
3) Can demonstrate at least one assertive behavior.

Recommended References
"Aggression as a Response," by Vallory G. Lathrop. *Perspectives in Psychiatric Care*, Sept.-Dec. 1978:202–205.
"Changing Behaviors: A Fun Approach that Works," by Kay M. Duffy. *RN*, December 1978:103–104.
"Mrs. Dowager: A Determinedly Disruptive Patient," by Mary T. Marks. *Nursing 73*, December 1973:17–19.
"The Violent Patient." *NCP Guide* #4:40, Nurseco, 1978.
"To Punish Herself, Laura Mutilated Her Body," by Karen R. Palermo. *Nursing 79*, June 1979:44–48.
"We Were No Match for 'Zorba the Greek'," by Darlene Rzepka. *Nursing 75*, September 1975:26–29.

© Margo Creighton Neal, 1980

NCP Guide No. **2:01** 3

The Patient with Alcoholism

Definition: A physiological dependence (addiction) on alcohol as a result of excessive use.

LONG TERM GOAL: The patient will be able to recognize and accept his addiction and to develop situational supports and coping mechanisms that reflect adaptation to a life style without alcohol.

General Considerations:
- In general hospitals, a patient with alcoholism is often admitted with another diagnosis which may or may not be related to use of alcohol. Excessive use can cause many physical problems such as: gastritis, chronic diarrhea, vitamin and nutritional deficiencies, disorders of neurological and cardiac systems, pancreatitis, fatty liver, cirrhosis, hypoglycemia.
- The **cause** of alcoholism is not known, but it seems to be affected by: (1) *social factors* (customs, attitudes towards drinking; amount of stress and tension in the community), and (2) the individual's *personality traits* (tend to be generally uneasy and dissatisfied with life; tend to excesses in areas such as work, sex, recreation; low frustration tolerance; dependence on others; poor ability to cope with stress).
- Alcohol depresses higher cortical functions, acts as a disinhibitor and tranquilizer and serves to reduce anxiety rapidly; excessive drinking is often the way a person copes with anxiety.
- Alcohol addiction often creates behavioral responses that are considered erratic, irresponsible, destructive. It may create a situation where the alcohol need is dominant and the purpose of living is to maintain alcohol intake.
- The **severity of withdrawal** symptoms is the direct result of the increased levels of acetaldehyde and decreased magnesium levels in the blood (breakdown products of alcohol).
- **General treatment measures** include vitamin and nutritional therapy, use of sedatives, tranquilizers, and/or Antabuse.
- **Preventive measures** include helping the patient learn (1) to tolerate psychological stress; (2) to do advance planning for anticipated painful events (surgery, separation from a loved one); and (3) to reduce social isolation.
- **Nursing responsibilities** include adequate treatment and maintenance of life functions during withdrawal, as well as teaching and support of preventative measures in those predisposed to alcoholism.

Specific Considerations, Potential Patient Outcomes, and Nursing Actions:

1) Maintenance of Body Functioning During

The patient will withdraw from the alcohol free of the complications of dehydration, electrolyte imbalance, nutritional imbalance; will verbally recognize and discuss his alcoholism as the cause of the withdrawal:
- know that the severity of withdrawal symptoms is related to the length & extent of drinking preceding the withdrawal period;

Withdrawal	—	complete cessation of use of alcohol is not necessary for the development of withdrawal symptoms; the beginning of withdrawal can be a reflection of diminished use in those who have developed a high tolerance and physical dependence; observe for withdrawal symptoms as early as 8 hours after cessation of drinking;
	—	withdrawal is a progressive process and involves four stages:

- Stage I   8 hours + after cessation: symptoms include mild tremors, nausea, nervousness, tachycardia, increased blood pressure, & diaphoresis.
- Stage II   symptoms include gross tremors, nervousness & hyperactivity, insomnia, anorexia, general weakness, disorientation, illusions, nightmares; auditory & visual hallucinations begin.
- Stage III   12-48 hours after cessation: symptoms include all those of Stages I and II, as well as severe hallucinations & grand mal seizures.
- Stage IV   occurs 3-5 days after cessation: symptoms include initial & continuing DTs (delirium tremens) which are characterized by confusion, severe psychomotor activity, agitation, sleeplessness, hallucinations, & uncontrolled & unexplained tachycardia at onset.

— control symptoms via PRN medication; take vital signs Q2H & report elevated ones to doctor;
— if pt. is agitated, confused, etc., stay with him; reassure that current symptoms are only result of his body responding to alcohol use, & that they are temporary; tell him he will regain control; use restraints only if absolutely necessary;
— deal with hallucinations by reinforcing reality; speak to pt. slowly in a calm voice; provide a quiet environment; stay with pt. until the frightening symptoms have decreased;
— ensure a daily fluid intake of at least 2500 cc's orally (unless contraindicated; check with Dr.); offer favorite juices Q2H during waking hours; prevent excessive coffee or tea intake;
— identify pt.'s food preferences; provide frequent small feedings or in-between meal snacks of high-protein foods; involve pt. in food-related planning; give multivitamin & mineral supplements as ordered;
— provide physical care advocated for additional diseases/conditions pt. may have;
— keep pt. ambulatory as much as possible; if necessary, walk with pt. several times a day; help to bathroom, rather than providing bed pan or urinal.

2) Psychosocial Adjustment (to Life without Alcohol)

The patient will discuss and develop the use of coping mechanism other than alcohol to deal with the stress and strain of daily life:
— sit & visit with pt. at least twice daily; your presence will say s/he is not being rejected for any behavior;
— discuss your observations of pt.'s behavior with him, helping him develop insight re: its relation with alcohol intake;

- in an accepting, non-judgmental way, discuss pt.'s use of alcohol with him; provide information as he wants and asks for it; seek help of a psychiatric nurse or mental health specialist if you cannot do this;
- recognize & share with pt. that a lifestyle without alcohol is a major loss to him (see NCPG #1:31, "Response to Loss. . ."); anticipate what this may mean & help him plan adaptive ways to compensate for the loss;
- do not punish or reprimand pt. for failures or nonresponse to your suggestions/interventions; (punishment serves only to give pt. fuel for continuing to deal with failure or rejection by drinking) ignore it, but do praise *any* positive responses;
- have pt. make decisions about daily care in hospital; involve him in some type of occupational therapy, anything in which he can achieve some measure of success (helps increase self-confidence and self-esteem);
- provide opportunities to decrease social isolation & improve social skills (meal times, pt. groups, recreation periods); calmly, gently, point out unacceptable behavior such as manipulative ones (see NCPG #1:20, "The Patient Displaying Manipulation"); reinforce positive social behaviors (e.g. initiating friendly conversations); praise all efforts at participation in activities;
- if pt. on Antabuse therapy, read literature & then explain effects that develop with ingestion of alcohol (severe nausea & vomiting, flushed face, rapid pulse and respirations, drop in BP);
- arrange for pt. & family to attend group counseling sessions, if available in hospital, to discuss feelings, problems, changing behaviors, pressures, sources of support, etc.;
- discuss AA with pt.; offer to arrange for a member to come & see pt. & encourage him to accept; provide information about other types of therapy available, e.g. local mental health clinics.

3) Functional, Situational Support Systems

The patient will accept the support of others; will discuss with them how they can help him live without alcohol:
- hold weekly health team conferences to discuss aspects of alcoholism, share feelings & responses to caring for an alcoholic pt., & to coordinate care; explain that it is normal for staff to feel frustrated (angry, guilty, rejecting, anxious) when caring for alcoholic pts.; staff often feel they have failed if a pt. is readmitted in an alcoholic state after they had discharged him "improved"; include a psych. nurse or other mental health specialist;
- request inservice education programs, films, literature, etc. on alcoholism;
- permit family to express their anger at pt.'s exacerbations; listen to & support them; put family in touch with a community group where consistent support & help are available, e.g. Al Anon (family group of AA);
- invite a member of AA &/or Al Anon to a staff conference to share their aims, approaches, etc., or go to a meeting with a colleague.

Discharge Planning and Teaching Objectives/Outcomes
1. (Patient/Family/Significant Other) Has a contact with Alcoholics Anonymous, Al Anon and/or other community mental health group.
2) Verbalizes an understanding of and expects to participate in a daily program of balanced food and fluid intake, rest, exercise, and recreation.
3) Can state the actions and side effects of current medications; has an adequate supply to take with him.
4) Has at least one plan to help decrease social isolation and strengthen new behaviors.

Recommended References
"Alcoholism" (and other publications). National Council on Alcoholism, Inc., 2 Park Avenue, New York, NY 10016.
"Assessing Alcoholic Patients," by E. Heinemann and N. Estes. *American Journal of Nursing*, May 1976:785–789.
"Helping the Alcoholic Cope With . . . Sobriety," by Mary Ann Boyson. *RN*, July 1975:37.
"Maternal Alcoholism and the Fetal Alcohol Syndrome," by Barbara Luke. *American Journal of Nursing*, December 1977:1924–1926.
"Rehabilitating the Problem Drinker," by J. Carroll and M. Synigal. *Nursing Digest*, Fall, 1976:44–46.
"Rehabilitation for Alcoholics," by Joyce Ditzler. *American Journal of Nursing*, November 1976:1772–1774.
"Responses to Loss: the Grief and Mourning Process." NCP Guide #1:31, 2nd ed., Nurseco, 1980.
"The Alcoholic Surgical Patient," Nursing Grand Rounds, *Nursing '77*, May 1977:56–61.
"The Value of Life," Nursing Grand Rounds, *Nursing '79*, July 1979:30–37.

© Margo Creighton Neal, 1980

The Patient Manifesting Anger

Definition: A strong feeling of displeasure, usually of antagonism.

LONG TERM GOAL: The patient will use realistic and self-protective (assertive) behavior to express his displeasure.

General Considerations:
— **Each angry outburst should be reviewed** with a goal of improving patient care by identifying situations which contributed to the outburst and by evaluating and revising interventions.
— **Nursing assessment** includes awareness of the behavioral manifestations of anger which include:
  — abusive verbal language;
  — constant negative verbalizations regarding hospital and staff;
  — refusal to participate in care;
  — refusal to eat or drink;
  — refusal to be dependent on staff;
  — throwing food or objects;
  — removal of treatment equipment from self (e.g. pulling out IV);
  — silence.
— **Nursing responsibilities** include assessment of the anger-provoking situation for cause and effect as well as assessment of the patient's usual coping behaviors in order to recognize and support those that are adaptive and positive.

Specific Considerations, Potential Patient Outcomes, and Nursing Actions:

1) Immediate Response to Recognition of Expressed Anger

The patient will eliminate the physically harmful and attacking expressions of anger; will express anger assertively rather than aggressively:
— tell the pt. you will prevent any further expression of anger that is physically harmful in nature;
— spend time with the pt.; ask him what the anger is about; if s/he refuses to answer, just sit with him while he is silent;
— praise any pt. efforts to put the anger into words & share the causes with you;
— be aware that a pt.'s anger is usually not meant for you personally, so do not respond defensively.

2) Restoration to Adaptive Coping

The patient will be able to discuss situations that provoke angry feelings; will be able to verbalize both positive and negative feelings related to angry outbursts:
— invite the pt. to participate in own care & to discuss feelings about the hospitalization;
— involve the pt. in own care on a continuing basis; ask him to do specific parts while you do others; discuss the results of this shared responsibility with him;
— continue to spend time daily conversing with the pt.; direct the conversation towards those aspects of the illness for which s/he has the most negative feelings; use open-ended questions;
— spend time with pt.'s significant others explaining pt.'s need to have the opportunity to express both positive & negative feeling about what is happening to him;
— praise the efforts of others to accept the conversational expressions by the pt. of his negative feelings;
— praise staff & family efforts to support the pt. & to understand the pt.'s behavior without personalizing it.

Discharge Planning and Teaching Objectives/Outcomes
1) (Patient/Family/Significant Other) Can verbalize behavior or demands that trigger the physically harmful aspects of patient's anger.
2) Can describe the difference between the conversational expression of anger and physically harmful/forceful behavior.
3) Can share both positive and negative feelings about an individual experience.

Recommended References
"Dealing with Rage." Nursing Grand Rounds. *Nursing 75*, October, 1975:24–29.
"Hostility," by Sister M. Martha Kiening in Carlson, Carolyn and Blackwell, Betty *Behavioral Concepts and Nursing Intervention*, 2nd ed., Philadelphia: J.B. Lippincott Co., 1978:128–140.
"Mr. O'Brien's Beard," by Rosemaire Hogan. *American Journal of Nursing*, January 1977:61.
"Privacy," by Dorothy W. Bloch in Carlson and Blackwell, *Behavioral Concepts and Nursing Interventions*, 2nd ed., Philadelphia: J.B. Lippincott, Co., 1978:226–239.
"The Staff Called Mrs. Jepson's Care Plan 'Resocialization.' I Called It a Repressive Regimen," by Joan Schuettler. *Nursing 74*, August 1974:10–12.
"The Violent Patient." *NCP Guide* #4:40, Nurseco, 1979.
"Understanding Anger," by Derry Ann Moritz. *American Journal of Nursing*, January 1978:81–83.
"We Should Have Been Tougher with Emma . . . and Ourselves," by Deborah Roediger. *Nursing 77*, May 1977:48–49.

© Margo Creighton Neal, 1980

NCP Guide No. **4:36** 9

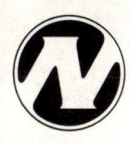

The Patient with an <u>Antisocial Personality</u>

Definition: A cluster of personality characteristics manifested by deeply ingrained, basically unsocialized behavior. Formerly known as sociopathic or psychopathic personality.

LONG TERM GOAL: The patient will recognize and observe limits in interactions with others.

General Considerations:

- <u>Characteristics</u>: The antisocial individual does not tolerate frustration, feels little guilt, and does not change behavior because of punishment. Though this person often has an outwardly pleasing, charming personality, s/he is loyal only to own self, has no close personal relationships, and "uses" or manipulates other people and events for own motives. There is a tendency to blame others for the same behavior; has never learned to give, only to take. The antisocial individual does not see self as mentally ill and infrequently presents self for treatment. Usually hospitalized for treatment of other disorders, to withdraw from alcohol or drugs, or as result of a court order for psychiatric evaluation or treatment. Described as selfish, irresponsible, impulsive and callous; repeatedly in conflict with society, and often with the law.
- <u>Treatment</u> usually consists of applying external controls to limit the acting-out behavior; antisocial behavior patterns are difficult to alter and respond poorly to treatment. Long-term psychotherapy has had the most success in changing behavior pattersn, but relatively few patients remain in psychotherapy because of expense, time involved, and poor motivation and insight.
- <u>Nursing responsibilities</u> include reinforcing reality, preventing manipulation of self and others by patient, protecting other patients and self from this patient and health-teaching as needed.

Specific Considerations, Potential Patient Outcomes and Nursing Actions:

1) Manipulation The patient will recognize and observe limits in interactions with others:
    - be aware that staff commonly experience uncomfortable feelings of anger, helplessness, frustration, defensiveness, etc. when working with these pts.; openly discussing and acknowledging these feelings with other staff can lead to control of them, thus making one less susceptible to being manipulated; refer to NCPG #1:29, "Manipulation;"
    - observe closely pt's. behavior & interactions with staff & other pts.; assess the meaning & understanding of the behavior to the pt. & validate with pt. & other staff; hold a staff conference to discuss, set & inform all staff of approaches & limits for this pt.; written care plans will provide the best means for consistency of approach on all three shifts;
    - be aware of other pts. who could easily be affected by pt. (used, hurt) & intervene PRN; work with both pts. on appropriate

- alternatives to respond to each other; if antisocial pt. refuses to cooperate, separate from rest of unit for time out; state firmly that limits will be set on behavior & that people & situations will not be used for one person's motives; make contract with pt. that states specific cause & effect, such as, "If you take Mr. H's cigarettes, you will not be allowed in the day room when he is there;" follow through on contract on all shifts; be consistent;
- review requests made by pt. with other staff before permission is granted or denied; do not make "on-the-spot" decisions if possible; remember that this pt. is often an expert at pitting one staff member against another (recreating the family triangle & s/he is the center of attention); staff must present a united front to the pt.;
- give attention to pt. when s/he is not manipulating; reinforce positive behavior; (often the only attention pt. gets, occurs after s/he "acts out" or manipulates); set reasonable goals with pt.; reinforce positive efforts to reach them;
- explanations, discussions should be short & simple as long, complex ones can be another aspect of manipulation;
- be aware that pt. may use tears, lies, threats to get what s/he wants; limits must be followed by all staff members & may be lifted as pt. shows s/he can handle responsibility;
- know that pt's. demands may be endless; be firm and, most important of all, be consistent.

2) Difficulty with Social Relationships

The patient will strengthen ability to relate to others in socially acceptable ways:
- assess & help pt. define problem areas in social relationships—e.g. blames others, lack of concern for others;
- encourage pt. to discuss this problem area in group therapy & to ask others why they reject him (if true);
- practice social skills, use role-playing; give positive reinforcement for positive behavior.

3) Acting Out or Violent Behavior

See NCPG #4:40, "The Patient Who is Violent."

Discharge Planning and Teaching Objectives/Outcomes:
1) (Patient and/or Family/Significant Other) Can cite some limits to interactions with others.
2) Has demonstrated ability to comply with social mores and to behave within socially acceptable limits at least part of the time (to an increasing amount)
3) Indicates a willingness to continue mental health therapy in some form that is presently available and potentially helpful.

Recommended References
"The Patient Displaying Manipulation," NCP Guides, #1:29, Nurseco, 1974.
"The Patient Who is Violent," NCP Guides, #4:40, Nurseco, 1978.
Psychiatric Nursing in the Hospital and the Community, 2nd edition, by Ann Burgess and Aaron Lazare, Englewood Cliffs, NJ: Prentice-Hall, Inc., 1976.
Therapeutic Approaches to the Care of the Mentally Ill, by David Bailey, Ed D. and Sharon Dreyer, RN, MSN, Philadelphia: F. A. Davis Co., 1977.

© Margo Creighton Neal, 1978

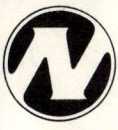

The Patient Experiencing Anxiety

Definition: An uncomfortable feeling or tension which can be vague and/or intense. It occurs as a reaction to some unconscious threat that the person is experiencing.

LONG TERM GOAL: The patient will be able to use anxiety as a motivation for change and not be immobilized by it.

General Considerations:
— **Anxiety serves as a force** that warns the individual about threatening situations.
— **Nursing assessment** includes knowledge of the behavioral and physiological manifestations of anxiety which include:

Behavioral Manifestations
— restlessness
— irritability
— rapid speech
— wringing of hands
— repetitious questioning
— inability to concentrate &/or understand explanations
— inability to retain information given
— somatic complaints
— inability to communicate
— putting call light on frequently
— disbelief of answers given

Physiological Manifestations
— increased blood pressure
— rapid breath and pulse
— muscular tension
— pounding heart
— dilated pupils
— perspiration
— gastric discomfort
— dry mouth
— headaches
— nausea
— dizziness
— trembling
— cold, clammy hands

— **Nursing responsibilities** include assessment of the level of anxiety:
  (1) **mild anxiety:** alertness; an ability to recognize anxiety as a warning signal; learning can occur at this level;
  (2) **moderate anxiety:** selective inattention; a decreased ability to communicate or perceive the environment unless it is pointed out; learning can still occur at this level but it must be directed;
  (3) **severe anxiety:** a drastically reduced ability to perceive and communicate details; the whole is perceived but the connection between details cannot be made; learning cannot occur at this level;
  (4) **panic:** any detail which is perceived is elaborated and distorted; the person is unable to communicate or function; learning cannot take place.
— **Nursing interventions** should be directed toward the support and enhancement of those behaviors that are adaptive, positive and have assisted in resolving anxiety in past situations. In the panic level, the only successful interventions are those designed to make the person comfortable and reassured.

Specific Considerations, Potential Patient Outcomes, and Nursing Actions:

1) **Immediate Response to Recognition of Anxious Behavior**

 The patient will be able to cope with the anxiety and reduce it at least one level:
 — spend at least five minutes with the pt. TID & try to convey a willingness to listen & be supportive;
 — encourage such coping mechanisms as talking, walking or crying;
 — give the pt. clear, concise explanations of what is going to occur; repeat as often as necessary;
 — do not overload the pt. with information; the pt. experiencing moderate to severe anxiety cannot retain or incorporate a great deal of data;
 — do not make demands of the pt.;
 — ask the pt. what you could do to make him feel more comfortable;
 — if pt. hyperventilating, have pt. take slow, deep breaths; ask him to focus on how his body feels on expiration; breathe with pt. to give support;
 — if pt. is in panic, stay with him, using physical touch PRN.

2) **Restoration to Adaptive Coping**

 The patient will be able to identify sources of his anxiety:
 — continue holding conversations with the pt.; increase the duration of each conversation but decrease the number of conversations per day;
 — help pt. identify those tensions & environmental factors that create a feeling of anxiety;
 — include the pt. in decisions about his care in order to create patient responsibility;
 — give careful explanations of what will occur; ask the pt. for questions or concerns s/he may have about these events;
 — encourage supportive family members to be patient since the pt. may not respond to them as before;
 — praise staff & family members who are able to maintain an environment for the pt. that allows him to gain an understanding of & control over the anxiety.

Discharge Planning and Teaching Objectives/Outcomes

1) (Patient/Family/Significant Other) Can verbalize the way in which s/he copes with severe anxiety.
2) Can list environmental factors that elicit anxiety.
3) Can discuss ways of keeping patient responses to anxiety at a mild or moderate level and successfully cope with it.

Recommended References

"Drugs: Tranquilizers." *NCP Guide* #3:47, Nurseco, 1977.
"Effects of Hospitalization: Part A Tension Producing Causes." *NCP Guide* #1:40, 2nd Ed., Nurseco, 1980.
"Mrs. Kluska Wasn't Difficult . . . She Was Impossible," by Eileen Jahubek. *Nursing 77*, July 1977:36–37.
"Panic: Three Easy Steps to Restoring Control," by Sally Langendoen. *RN*, December 1978:44–47.
"The Patient Needing Crises Intervention." *NCP Guide* #2:31, 2nd Ed., Nurseco, 1980.
"Teaching a Concept of Anxiety to Patients," by Dorothea R. Hays. *Nursing Research*, Spring 1961:108–113.

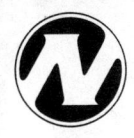

The Patient Experiencing a Body Image Disturbance

Definition: The inability of an individual to perceive and/or adapt to his body, or part of it, in a changed form.

LONG TERM GOAL: The patient will be able to manage his own life, make future goals and live with others while being aware that his body has changed.

General Considerations:
— **Body image** results from internal development as well as environmental experiences, including input from others, societal views, cultural practices, and previous experiences with persons whose bodies have been changed.
— **Nursing responsibilities** include an awareness of the causes of body image disturbances which are:
  (1) a real or anticipated loss of a body part and/or its usual functioning (colostomy, diabetes);
  (2) neurological disorders resulting in changes in locomotion and posture (e.g. paralysis);
  (3) metabolic or toxic disorders resulting in changes in body structure (e.g. kidney failure);
  (4) progressively-deforming disorders (e.g. arthritis);
  (5) acute dismemberment disorders (e.g. amputation, mastectomy);
  (6) personality development disorders (e.g. schizophrenia).
— **Nursing assessment** involves an awareness of the behavioral manifestations indicative of a body image disturbance and include:
  (1) refusal to continue functioning at any level, to believe any change has occurred and/or to look at altered body part;
  (2) inability to care for self or perform any activities of daily living;
  (3) withdrawal; hostility;
  (4) any behavior indicative of a response to a loss (e.g. shock, denial, anger); see NCPG #1:31, "Responses to Loss . . ."
— **Nursing interventions** should focus on assisting the patient to adapt to the loss which results from change and reinforcing those areas of continued daily functioning.

Specific Considerations, Potential Patient Outcomes, and Nursing Actions:

1) Immediate Response to Recognition of a Body Image Disturbance

The patient will be able to verbally state that a loss-change in body has occurred:
— provide openings for the pt. to express feelings by validating your observations & feelings with him (e.g. "You look down in the dumps; how are things going for you today?" or "You seem upset/sad. Are you?"); be a good listener & accept what pt. verbalizes; if s/he expresses anger or hostile feelings, remember not to take them personally; s/he may be handling them in the only way possible;

- focus on the pt.'s feelings & deal with the presenting behavior, e.g. if s/he is denying a body change that has actually occurred, do not challenge the pt.;
- determine what the body image change means to the pt.; how does s/he think it will affect his life? If you think his perceptions are unrealistic, do not challenge them at this time; the best intervention you can provide is the opportunity for him to share these perceptions & feelings with you;
- accept any body changes you observe in the pt.; if pt. is repulsed or ashamed of physical changes, s/he will be watching the faces of others for negative signs;
- provide basic needs for pt.; s/he may be very dependent on staff at this time;
- let the pt. know that the feelings & concerns s/he is experiencing are normal & that you are there to listen to him as well as help him cope.

2) Restoration to Adaptive Coping

The patient will accept the body alterations and verbalize how these will affect job, family life, view of life:
- give positive reinforcement for pt.'s efforts to adapt; his behavior will indicate when he starts to accept alterations in his body (may ask questions; will start to look at the incision, dressings, etc.); accept, but do not support expressions of denial;
- if a prosthesis will be used, assist pt. in his choice by providing information & arranging for a visit by someone from Colostomy Club, Reach for Recovery, or other appropriate group; let pt. determine time of visit, but try to arrange it as soon as possible;
- involve pt. in self care activities; begin slowly & add new activities one at a time; reinforce any efforts to participate;
- include in nursing care plan pt.'s perception of what the body change means to him, the objectives & nursing actions prescribed; share plan with all care givers, including family;
- tell others how they can help pt. by listening, supporting reality, allowing expressions of anger, denial, & not challenging them; permitting pt. to cry & giving positive reinforcement for all pt.'s efforts to cope/adapt;
- praise these others for their efforts to help pt.;
- hold a team conference, include family if you wish, & share information on "The Grief and Mourning Process" & "Crisis Intervention" (NCPG's #2:31, 35) with each other; discuss what parts of these concepts apply to this pt. at this time; revise the care plan PRN.

Discharge Planning and Teaching Objectives/Outcomes
1) (Patient/Family/Significant Other) Can identify how body has changed.
2) Can verbalize the fact that sadness and other feelings related to the loss are normal and part of the grief and mourning process.
3) Can accept continued support and positive input from significant others.
4) Can utilize community resources such as Reach for Recovery, Colostomy Club, to provide ongoing support, reassurance, and assistance in recovery.

Recommended References
"Crisis Intervention: Adaptation to General Nursing." NCP Guide #2:35, 2nd Ed., Nurseco, 1980.
"How To Make The Most of Body Image Theory in Nursing Practice," by Joanne McCloskey. *Nursing '76,* May 1976:68–72.
"Reestablishing Body Image," by Elaine Smith et al. *American Journal of Nursing,* March 1977:445–447.
"Responses to Loss: The Grief and Mourning Process," NCP Guide #1:31, 2nd Ed., Nurseco, 1980.
"Symposium on the Concept of Body Image." *Nursing Clinics of North America,* Philadelphia: W. B. Saunders Company, December 1972:593–707.
"The Patient Needing Crisis Intervention." NCP Guide #2:31, 2nd Ed., Nurseco, 1980.

© Margo Creighton Neal, 1980

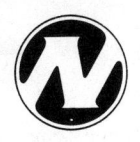

The Patient Adapting to Chronic Illness Role

Definition: Chronic illness is considered to be any impairment or deviation from normal health that has some of the following characteristics: 1) permanent, non-reversible, or residual impairment; 2) insidious onset; 3) requires a long period of supervision of care. Chronic illness role consists of behaviors related to the limitations imposed by the impairment or deviation from normal health and behaviors defined by society as appropriate to the limitations.

LONG TERM GOAL: The patient will adapt to limitations imposed by chronic illness; the patient will care for self and be as independent as possible; the patient will be motivated to retain whatever tasks and roles are possible.

General Considerations:
— Chronic illness involves a life-long period of treatment, usually with remissions and exacerbation of symptoms; this role is not seen by society as attractive or desired, and the patient is often separated from the well population during periods of exacerbation.
— Impairment requires special training for rehabilitation; the patient is expected to share in the planning and treatment process and to assume increasing responsibility for self-care.
— **Treatment goal** is to delay or control acute symptoms, promote comfort, maintain healthy bio-psycho-social systems, and rehabilitate to patient's full potential.
— **Nursing assessment** includes assessing the patient for behaviors associated with chronic illness role which may include:
  - hope, hopelessness
  - anger, frustration
  - depression
  - anxiety
  - fear of total disability or death
  - alterations in self-esteem
  - alterations in body-image
  - powerlessness
  - grief and mourning
  - feelings of being stigmatized, shame
  - instrumental and emotional dependence
  - motivation to retain roles and tasks.
— **Nursing responsibilities,** in addition to assessment, are to prevent deformities and complications, to motivate, to teach and support the patient and family in resuming self-care activities, and to refer patient for follow-up care and supervision.
— For additional information, refer to NCPGs #2:29, "Patient Experiencing a Body Image Disturbance," #5:32, "The Patient Experiencing a Threat to Self-Esteem," and #5:34, "The Patient Experiencing Powerlessness."

Specific Considerations, Potential Patient Outcomes, and Nursing Actions:

1) Immediate Response to Diagnosis of Chronic Illness

The patient experiences emotional support while reacting to diagnosis of chronic disease or disability; the patient participates in planning care, does as much self-care as limitations allow, and complies with treatment plan:
— assess pt. for behaviors of shock & disbelief, denial & other behaviors of loss; listen & give emotional support, accepting the pt.'s need to cope with the situation at his own pace; accept pt.'s denial at this time but do not support it (see NCPG #1:24, "The Patient Manifesting Denial");
— protect pt. from injury caused by denying or ignoring limitations; strive to prevent complications & deformities (see NCPGs #2:45, "The Hazards of Immobility" & #1:42, "Effects of Hospitalization: Part C: Prolonged Confinement");
— encourage pt. to participate in planning own care & to do as much self-care as limitations of chronic disease or disability will allow; be aware that pt. may become very dependent on first hearing diagnosis;
— assess pt. & family for knowledge of chronic disease process, treatment plan, treatments, medications, & for feelings & concerns; give positive reinforcement for knowledge & for cooperation with treatment plan;
— offer brief explanations if requested; wait until initial grief & mourning period is over to begin health teaching;
— be aware of adaptive & maladaptive behaviors associated with loss; assess pt.'s behaviors & support adaptive ones; refer to NCPG #1:31, "Responses to Loss;"
— know that pt. is in a state of conflict at forced dependence imposed by limitations with threat to usual lifestyle & self-esteem; maintain hope for rehabilitation without supporting false hopes or unrealistic goals.

2) Adaptation to Chronic Disease or Disability

The patient begins to recognize and cope with limitations; the patient becomes committed to rehabilitation program:
— emphasize pt.'s assets & strengths; give positive reinforcement with praise & attention as pt. begins to show progress & commitment to treatment plan & rehabilitation program;
— set short-term goals with pt. in order to increase ability to be independent in ADL (activities of daily living); encourage pt. to do independent therapeutic exercises & ROM (see NCPG #1:47, "Range of Motion Exercises") as ordered by physician & physical therapist;
— know that participation in ADL & exercise program is essential to restore motivation & optimism in pt., as well as to retain muscle tone & ROM;
— be a creative problem solver with the pt. & the health care team to assist the pt. to use self-help devices when s/he has difficulty performing an activity; self-help devices may include adaptive equipment for mobility, personal care aids, communication, writing & typewriting aids (see NCPG #5:47, "Problem Solving");

- assess for readiness to learn about disease process, treatment plan, medication & prognosis; health teach pt. & family as indicated; see NCPGs #1:49 & 50, "Teaching Patients;"
- assess hobbies & pastimes to encourage socialization & to avoid boredom & sensory monotony;
- be aware that persons with chronic illness or disability are still sexual beings; assist pt. to deal with sexual concerns by health teaching, counseling or referral to a counselor who specializes in sexual counseling for the handicapped;
- assist pt. to retain roles & tasks as much as possible within existing limitations;
- know that chronic illness has vacillations between remission & control of illness with a decrease in symptoms, & exacerbations & extension of illness with increase in symptoms;
- be prepared to support pt. emotionally & with comfort measures & treatment of acute symptoms during exacerbations; pt. may fear further disability, pain, increased dependence, & death; see NCPG #1:28, "The Patient Experiencing Fear."

3) Referral to Follow-up Care and Supervision

The patient receives referrals for follow-up care and supervision:
- begin planning for discharge on the day of admission; the pt.'s functional potential should be estimated & continually assessed so that discharge plans can be made by health care team;
- give pt. increased support when discharge is near; many pts. experience some "separation anxiety" & have concerns about leaving hospital;
- assess attitudes & concerns of family members; family therapy may be indicated for rejection & avoidance;
- send ADL assessment home or to extended care facility so that visiting nurse or staff will be able to reinforce independent progress in ADL;
- advise pt. & family of Rehabilitation Services Administration which provides diagnosis, treatment, counseling, training, & placement services to help the pt. towards vocational objectives;
- inform pt. of voluntary & self-help groups in community;
- tell pt. & family about the Directory of National Information Sources on Handicapping Conditions and Related Services (contains abstracts and addresses of 270 organizations offering services, information, and resources to handicapped individuals); obtain a copy from Superintendent of Documents, Government Printing Office, Washington, DC 20420.

Discharge Planning and Teaching Objectives/Outcomes

1) (Patient/Family/Significant Other) Can describe in own words chronic disease process and medical treatment plan, including action and side effects of medication, exercise program, diet, etc.

2) Can identify symptoms or side effects of medications which should be reported to physician right away.
3) Can describe rehabilitation program and adapt to limitations of chronic illness.
4) Knows appropriate support services and how to contact (e.g., social worker, rehabilitation services, self-help groups, etc.)

Recommended References

"The Chronic Mentally Ill in the Community—Case Management Models," by J. Lanoil. *Psychosocial Rehabilitation Journal,* Spring/Summer 1980: 1–60.
"Disability, Home Care, and the Care Taking Role in Family Life," by A.J. Davis. *Journal of Advanced Nursing,* September 1980: 475–484.
"Effects of Hospitalization: Part C: Prolonged Confinement." *NCP Guide #1:42,* 2nd Ed., Nurseco, 1980.
"Hazards of Immobility." *NCP Guide #2:45,* 2nd Ed., Nurseco, 1980.
"Mutual Withdrawal . . . the Powerful Effects of Nursing Relationships on Very Difficult and Intractable Patient Behavior," by A.T. Slavensky et al. *Perspectives in Psychiatric Care,* September/October, 1980: 194–203.
"The Patient Experiencing a Body Image Disturbance." *NCP Guide #2:29,* 2nd Ed., Nurseco, 1980.
"The Patient Experiencing Fear." *NCP Guide #1:28,* 2nd Ed., Nurseco, 1980.
"The Patient Experiencing Powerlessness." *NCP Guide #5:34,* Nurseco, 1981.
"The Patient Experiencing a Threat to Self Esteem." *NCP Guide #5:32,* Nurseco, 1981.
"The Patient Manifesting Denial." *NCP Guide #1:24,* 2nd Ed., Nurseco, 1980.
"Political Advocacy for the Chronic Mental Disabled," by C. Bellamy et al. *Psychosocial Rehabilitation Journal,* Spring/Summer 1980: 7–11.
"Problem Solving." *NCP Guide #5:47,* Nurseco, 1981.
"Psychosocial Aspects of Chronic Illness in Children," by J. Assacs et al. *Journal of School Health,* August 1980: 318–321.
"Range of Motion Exercises." *NCP Guide #1:47,* 2nd Ed., Nurseco, 1980.
"Responses to Loss: The Grief and Mourning Process." *NCP Guide #1:31,* 2nd Ed., Nurseco, 1980.
"Teaching Patients: General Suggestions." *NCP Guide #1:49,* 2nd Ed., Nurseco, 1980.
"Teaching Patients: Specific Plan for Skills and Procedures." *NCP Guide #1:50,* 2nd Ed., Nurseco, 1980.

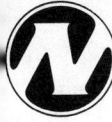

The Patient Experiencing Confusion

Definition: A quality or state of being perplexed. It is the inability to comprehend and/or integrate words or events; may be of a temporary or permanent nature.

LONG TERM GOAL: The patient will be able to maintain touch with reality as much as possible.

General Considerations:
— **Confusion occurs** as a result of trauma, rapid change, infectious and metabolic disturbances, neurologic conditions, drug intoxication, cardiac and respiratory disturbances, and drug and alcohol withdrawal.
— **Nursing assessment** includes an awareness of the manifestations of confusion which include:
  — inability or vague identification of time, place, person;
  — appears drowsy most of the time;
  — decreased or no attention span;
  — recent memory is impaired;
  — inability to retain information given;
  — more confused at night than in daytime;
  — restless, aimless motions;
  — physical assault;
  — does not make eye contact for any period of time.
— **Nursing responsibilities** include assessment of the physiological state of functioning of the patient in order to differentiate between physiologically-induced confusion and psychologically and/or environmentally-induced confusion.
— **Nursing interventions** should reflect the causative factors. If the confusion is physiologically based, then nursing care must focus on the restoration of adaptive, physiological functioning; behavioral techniques can enhance the recovery but the basic physiological disturbance must be cleared up.

Specific Considerations, Potential Patient Outcomes, and Nursing Actions:

1) Immediate Response to Recognition of Confusion

The patient will recover from the physiologically or environmentally/psychologically-induced confusion and regain as much contact with reality as possible:
— direct nursing care to the support of those physiological functions that are intact; give appropriate nursing care, & follow medical orders for treatment of the dysfunction;
— always address the pt. by name & say who you are; the pt. may hear & understand you even if s/he does not acknowledge you;

- be consistent in informing the pt. what you are going to do; do not assume s/he is so confused that s/he will not understand;
- consistently involve the pt. in decision making & activity;
- reduce the amount of sensory overload/deprivation the pt. is experiencing: *for overload*: turn down lights or reduce noise of equipment; try to schedule nursing care activities so the pt. will have quiet times; *for deprivation*: have a staff member or another less confused pt. spend time with this pt., especially at mealtimes; seat the pt. with others or encourage familiar & positive visitors; whenever you are near the pt., touch him, say hello, bring pt. out of room into areas where s/he will have access to additional sensory stimuli;
- utilize appropriate safety measures to prevent injury to the pt. & others.

2) Restoration to Reality

The patient will maintain contact with reality as much as possible and will be aware of the need for assistance.
- praise the pt. for efforts at being with others & involved with the environment;
- be honest with the pt., don't just go along with his "reality," & don't encourage a denial of the confusion;
- avoid letting the pt. ramble, bring the conversation back to reality;
- use clear concise statements & questions; speak slowly & allow plenty of time for the pt. to answer; do not rush him;
- have pt. keep familiar objects with him, i.e., clock, own sleepwear, pictures of family, friends;
- have family members or friends share "old times" with the pt.;
- support & praise the pt.'s efforts to maintain conversation & reality-oriented behavior, encourage staff & the family to praise pt. for these efforts.

Discharge Planning and Teaching Objectives/Outcomes

1) (Patient/Family/Significant Other) Can identify time, place and person and is able to maintain a conversation that is indicative of being in touch with reality.
2) Can identify the continued partial or complete confusion and make arrangements for appropriate home care or placement.

Recommended References

"Breaking Through the Cobwebs of Confusion in the Elderly," by Carolyn Stevens. *Nursing 74*, August 1974:41–48.
"Caring for the Confused or Delirious Patient," by Gordon Trochman. *American Journal of Nursing*, September 1978:1495–1499.
"The Aged Patient: Chronic Organic Brain Syndrome." *NCP Guide #4:34*, Nurseco, 1978.
"The Aged Patient: Common Behaviors." *NCP Guide #2:26*, 2nd Ed., Nurseco, 1980.
"The Aged Patient: Reality Orientation." *NCP Guide #3:33*, Nurseco, 1977.
"The Aged Patient: Resocialization." *NCP Guide #3:34*, Nurseco, 1977.
"The Aged Patient: Transition to Communal Living." *NCP Guide #2:27*, 2nd Ed., Nurseco, 1980.
"The Confused Patient: Assessing Mental Status," by Marilyn Dodd. *American Journal of Nursing*, September 1978:1501–1503.
"The Confused Patient: Responses in Critical Care Units," by Margaret Adams et al. *American Journal of Nursing*, September 1978:1504–1512.
"The Confused Patient: Out of Touch with Reality," by Olive Wilkinson. *American Journal of Nursing*, September 1978:1492–1494.

The Patient Needing Crisis Intervention

Definition: Crisis intervention refers to those approaches used to restore a patient to a state of emotional equilibrium from one of disequilibrium (the crisis state).

LONG TERM GOAL: The patient will achieve adaptive resolution of the crisis; will return to his usual job/roles with a realistic perception of what has occurred and with adequate coping mechanisms.

General Considerations:
- Read NCPG #2:35, "Crisis Intervention: Adaptation to General Nursing."
- In a non-psychiatric setting, the major loss or hazard is often situational: what brought the patient in, e.g. physical illness, trauma. Additional losses may include: loss of job, of independence, of usual role functioning, of usual living style (as in transfer to a nursing home).
- **Common manifestations** of a crisis include:
  - overwhelming feelings of helplessness, hopelessness
  - feelings of inability to cope anymore
  - feelings of loss of control over own life
  - decreased ability to carry out own activities of daily living
  - increased dependence on others
  - high anxiety; may develop into a panic state
  - inability to work and/or carry out usual roles
  - increased somatic complaints
- **Nursing responsibilities** focus initially on adequate assessment:
  - assessment of the patient and his current situation will tell you if the patient is in an actual crisis or in a hazardous situation. If the former, the objective is to help the patient achieve adaptive resolution of the crisis; if the latter, the objective is to prevent a crisis from occurring.
  - although hazardous situations create stress for *all* people, why do they develop into a crisis for some and not for others? This has to do with the presence or absence of balancing factors; assessment of these factors is essential.

Specific Considerations, Potential Patient Outcomes, and Nursing Actions:

1) Immediate Response to Recognition of an Actual or Potential Crisis

The patient will verbalize what s/he is experiencing; will express a feeling of decreasing anxiety; will identify those components that are most anxiety-producing:
— read NCPG #1:22, "The Patient Experiencing Anxiety";
— ask the pt. what is happening to him right now (scared? afraid? panicky? hopeless?) what occurred to make him feel like this? (accident? new diagnosis? new equipment in room?);
— allow pt. to respond at length & in detail to your questions; do not challenge any statements; try to determine exactly what is *most* threatening to him; listen & encourage pt. to keep talking;
— determine the real/anticipated pt. loss/losses involved; assess behavior in light of the Grief & Mourning Process (see NCP Guide #1:31, "Responses to Loss . . .");
— change the environment to reduce impact of the hazard, e.g. change room, allow family to stay, etc.;
— ask the pt. what you could do to make him feel better right now; if at all possible, provide it;
— provide basic needs; pt. may be very dependent in ADL; allow this dependency to occur for the immediate time;
— when you leave room, tell pt. when you will be back & return when you say you will;
— share information with pt. re: tests, procedures, etc.; tell him what he can expect (will help decrease feelings of anxiety, hopelessness);
— when the pt.'s behavior indicates that s/he is beginning to adapt or cope (begins to ask questions, focus on reality), support & reinforce reality; share with pt. how you see it; ask him to clarify or validate your perceptions.

2) Restoration to Adaptive Coping

The patient will express feelings of decreased hopelessness and helplessness; will regain a degree of control over own life; will develop alternate solutions to cope with current problem:
— continue to give pt. as much information as s/he wants to know about hospitalization, treatment, therapy; ask for feedback to ensure pt. understanding;
— help pt. increase independence in ADL: involve in self-care, slowly at first, then gradually adding more activities;
— provide opportunities for pt. to make decisions about daily care (this gives pt. some control over own life); praise pt. for making decisions, for coping with current stress, for helping self to feel better;
— help pt. brainstorm alternate solutions to current problem & look at the pros & cons of each one; don't tell pt. what to do, but ask if one of the solutions could possibly work for him;
— assess pt.'s perceptions of what has happened to him & correct any misperceptions;

— encourage pt. to share feelings, perceptions, new coping options, etc. with family/significant others; encourage them, in turn, to support pt.; explain to all the importance of the three balancing factors in pt. maintenance of equilibrium;
— check the effectiveness of pt.'s new coping options by asking what s/he would do if confronted with a situation similar to the one s/he has just experienced; reinforce positive adaptation & coping & teach PRN.

Discharge Planning and Teaching Objectives/Outcomes
1) (Patient/Family/Significant Other) Has a realistic expectation of what occurred and can verbalize what patient was feeling at the time.
2) Has adequate situational supports in the form of family, friends, job.
3) Can verbalize at least three options s/he can use to cope with stress.
4) Has name of a community resource to go to if s/he finds self in another hazardous situation with which s/he cannot cope.

Recommended References
"Crisis Intervention: Adaptation to General Nursing." NCP Guide #2:35, 2nd Ed., Nurseco, 1980.
"Crisis Intervention in Acute Care Areas," by Sandra H. Huenzi and Mary V. Fenton, *American Journal of Nursing*, May 1975:830–834.
"Responses to Loss: the Grief and Mourning Process." NCP Guide #1:31, 2nd Ed., Nurseco, 1980.
"Symposium on Crisis Intervention," *Nursing Clinics of North America*, Philadelphia: W.B. Saunders Company, March 1974:1–96.

© Margo Creighton Neal, 1980

The Patient Manifesting Denial

Definition: The manifestation of a person's inability or refusal to consciously acknowledge any thought, feeling, wish, or need of an external occurrence, or the threat of an occurrence.

LONG TERM GOAL: The patient will be able to interact with the environment in such a way that s/he maintains integrity and control but is not harmful to self.

General Considerations:
- **Denial occurs** as an unconscious effort to resolve emotional conflict and reduce the related anxiety. It occurs most often as a response to some threat to the status quo, i.e. trauma, illness, major life changes.
- **Nursing assessment** includes awareness of the manifestations of denial which include:
  - disbelief of diagnosis, symptoms, progress and/or information given;
  - changes information in such a way that it can be termed distorted;
  - refuses to discuss the hospitalization, surgery, trauma, or diagnosis;
  - refuses to participate in self care, either total body care or one aspect of care, i.e. colostomy care;
  - refuses medication, food, and/or all treatments;
  - refuses to follow recommendations such as bedrest, positioning, when these activities do not produce any increase in discomfort and may actually be more comfortable.
- **Nursing responsibilities** include monitoring activities of the patient so that the efforts at denial do not cause the patient harm, and supporting any patient efforts to understand what is happening to him.
- **Nursing interventions** should reflect the recognition of the patient's need to deal with the new situation at his own pace as long as this pace and method are not harmful.

Specific Considerations, Potential Patient Outcomes, and Nursing Actions:

1) Immediate Response to Recognition of Denial

   The patient will eliminate the physically harmful aspects of the denial:
   - relieve anxiety through the establishment of a trusting relationship;
   - spend time with the pt., listen to him verbalize about areas of his life other than the focus of denial;
   - identify & support the pt. using other coping mechanisms, i.e. talking, crying;
   - attempt to identify the most threatening aspects of reality by observing when the pt. reacts the most intensely, i.e. pt. is on a thousand calorie diet & has the family bring in fattening food;

- do not support the denial but give pt. adequate care & converse with him frequently; do not avoid him;
- attempt to introduce realities slowly by beginning with the least threatening part of the reality, e.g. pt. refuses to begin looking at or caring for his colostomy; begin by discussing diet & then gradually move the conversation into discussing diet for colostomy pts.

2) Restoration to Adaptive Coping

The patient will accept the change and handle self care without supervision:
- continue to involve the pt. in own care by planning time, place & kind of care with him;
- praise & encourage any interest the pt. shows in knowing more about the change/illness;
- praise the pt.'s efforts in caring for self and/or beginning recognition of reality;
- help the pt. express angry and/or sad feelings by using open-ended questions, listening & spending time with him daily;
- spend time with significant others (SOs) to explain to them what is happening to the pt., and what they can do to assist & support the pt.'s positive efforts to cope;
- help other staff & SOs realize the importance of refraining from chastising the pt. &/or family when they are using denial to cope.

Discharge Planning and Teaching Objectives/Outcomes
1) (Patient/Family/Significant Other) Can discuss the positive and negative aspects of the change/illness.
2) Can follow those aspects of daily regimen that maintain life.
3) Can accept responsibility for possible effects of noncompliance with recommended regimen.

Recommended References
"Analogy: Weapon Against Denial," by Margaret S. Wacker. *American Journal of Nursing*, January 1974:71–73.
"Denial of Illness," by Sister M. Martha Kiening, in Carlson, Carolyn and Blackwell, Betty. *Behavioral Concepts and Nursing Interventions*, 2nd Ed., Philadelphia: J.B. Lippincott, Co., 1978:211–225.
"Mrs. Vinson Didn't Want Our Help," by Rhonda Lester. *Nursing 78*, August 1978:37–39.
"Solving the Riddle of Loss: 'Depression' and Other Responses." Filmstrips available from Nurseco, PO Box 145, Pacific Palisades, CA 90272.

© Margo Creighton Neal, 1980

The Patient Experiencing Dependency

Definition: A person's reliance on another person, persons, or things for continual support, reassurance and the meeting of needs.

LONG TERM GOAL: The patient will be interdependent, i.e. will rely on self and others.

General Considerations:
- **Dependency** is a passive means of control used to achieve one's desires for attention and input.
- **Confinement** in non-home like settings such as the hospital, extended care facility, etc., causes some dependency to occur and increases already existent dependency.
- **Nursing assessment** includes awareness of the manifestations of dependency which include:
  - refusal to participate in own care;
  - constantly asking staff to do for the patient what the patient is capable of doing for self;
  - asking staff to come into the room frequently;
  - constantly telling staff verbally and through behavior that s/he is "helpless" and unable to do anything alone;
  - refusal to learn new ways of caring for an altered self;
  - refusal and/or inability to make any decisions;
  - asking not to be transferred out of specialty units, eg. CCU, ICU.
- **Nursing responsibilities** include assessment of the patient's usual coping behaviors, and the length of time and extent of the dependency.

Specific Considerations, Potential Patient Outcomes, and Nursing Actions:

1) Immediate Response to Recognition of Dependency

    The patient will perform at least one activity independently:
    - attempt to identify the source of the dependency:
      a) ongoing lifelong style of coping; or
      b) environmentally stimulated: has the hospitalization decreased and/or removed so much of the pt.'s control that s/he has turned to dependency as a means of coping?
    - do not criticize or openly acknowledge the dependent behavior;
    - after careful explanation to the pt., set limits on the amount & type of dependent behavior that will be tolerated by the staff;
    - give frequent, intermittent attention at times other than when the pt. asks for something;
    - state when you will be back, return then or send someone else;

NCP Guide No. **1:25** **30**

		— praise any independent behaviors;
		— explain to the pt. that you will not allow him to be so dependent, because you respect him & realize that he was able to do things for himself prior to hospitalization, & now you do not want to take this independence away.
2)	Restoration to Adaptive Coping	The patient will identify needs which s/he can meet independently and needs with which s/he needs assistance:
		— begin participation slowly & start with one activity only: eg., have the pt. wash own face, or hold something for you; praise efforts if s/he participates, but don't make an issue out of it;
		— be supportive of & praise all independent efforts; if dependency is a lifelong pattern, you may not be able to change it but only set limits on the extent;
		— plan the nursing care with the pt., have the pt. make some decisions, but start with one or two decisions, not all of them;
		— give careful explanation about the pt.'s need to be more independent to family & significant others (SOs); tell them that they can be most helpful by getting the pt. to do some things for himself, & then praising these efforts;
		— praise the efforts of the SOs when they assist the pt. to be independent.

Discharge Planning and Teaching Objectives/Outcomes
1) (Patient/Family/Significant Other) Can verbalize those areas where s/he can care for self and those areas where s/he needs assistance.
2) Can perform activities of daily living without constant attention.

Recommended References
"Caring for the Totally Dependent Patient." Nursing Grand Rounds. *Nursing 76*, July 1976:38–43.
"Giving the Patient an Active Role," by Tryon and Leonard in Skipper and Leonard, *Social Interaction and Patient Care*, Philadelphia: J.B. Lippincott, Co., 1965.
"Operant Conditioning in Chronic Illness," by Fowler et. al. *American Journal of Nursing*, June 1969:1226.
"Tad Appeared Helpless . . . Yet He Was Controlling Us," by Sherry L. Watkins. *Nursing 78*, June 1978:62–64.
"The Work of Getting Well," by Catherine Norris. *American Journal of Nursing*, October 1969:2118.

© Margo Creighton Neal, 1980

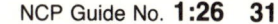

The Patient Experiencing Depression

Definition: An alteration in mood, usually related to a loss, and characterized by sadness, pessimism, despondence, hopelessness, and emptiness. It can also be aggression turned inward or the internalization of angry feelings.

LONG TERM GOAL: The patient will be able to talk positively and negatively about the loss, resume management of own life, and plan future goals.

General Considerations:
- **Depression is a response** to a real or perceived failure and/or a significant loss. See NCPG #1:31, "Responses to Loss." When resolution of the failure or loss is not complete, or complicated by additional failures or losses, the person will think that things cannot change and will "give up."
- **Nursing assessment** includes observing the patient for *behavioral manifestations of depression:* (1) stares off into space; (2) apathy (limited or no interest in self, others, or environment); (3) decreased initiative; (4) inability to concentrate; (5) decreased activity; (6) poor appetite; (7) complains of being, and looks, sad or tired all the time; (8) difficulty in getting to sleep at night and/or getting up in am; (9) feels sorry for self; (10) crying; and (11) withdrawal.
- **Nursing responsibilities** include an awareness of the difference between neurotic depression, described here, and psychotic depression (see NCP Guide #3:35, "The Patient Experiencing Depression (Psychiatric)"); an awareness of crisis intervention theory and practice, and an awareness of the signs and symptoms associated with suicidal risks. The focus of the nurse is on assisting the patient to regain control over own life and to express feelings s/he is experiencing.

Specific Considerations, Potential Patient Outcomes, and Nursing Actions:

1) Immediate Response to Recognition of Depression

The patient will verbally express feelings related to the painful event (i.e. failure and/or loss):
- make frequent, intermittent contact with the pt., both verbal & non-verbal;
- give attention consistently, even when the pt. is unwilling and/or unable to converse with you; this approach will establish you as an interested, caring person (depressed patients usually feel alone & worthless; a belief that someone is interested in & cares about them is the most helpful intervention);
- involve the pt. in self care & activities of daily living; start with one activity & gradually add others;
- suggest to the physician the use of anti-depressants, if you feel it is indicated;
- explore with pt. how s/he feels about listening to others' feelings (often people who have problems tolerating their own feelings tend to feel overwhelmed with others' feelings); practice sharing feelings of being overwhelmed & setting limits on listening to problems.

2) Restoration to Adaptive Coping

The patient will demonstrate the ability to carry out self care activities that are not physiologically impaired, make future plans and plan for discharge:
- continue to spend time with the pt. daily;
- use open-ended questions to elicit the pt.'s expression of feelings: e.g. "You look sad today. What is it that makes you feel this way?" acknowledge & reinforce any expression of feelings;
- do not tell the pt. s/he is not as sad or depressed as s/he feels; this approach only serves to reinforce the feeling that no one understands;
- make sure that everyone is aware of their responsibility for not chastizing the pt. when s/he is feeling sad;
- praise the pt. for any involvement in self care or other activities; encourage staff & significant others to praise pt. for these efforts;
- help pt. do things for self (many depressed pts. become dependent on others, but activity usually helps them to feel better);
- assist staff in their efforts to draw out the pt.; direct them to pay attention to him as much as possible;
- help pt. focus on meaning of loss, somatic symptoms, feelings tone: "You've had a hard time lately and you're learning to deal with your feelings." "You've lost functioning and you're going through grief and mourning."
- give positive reinforcement to reality & realistic expectations;
- identify problem areas & work out alternatives with pt.; take care to consider individual preferences & needs;
- assess areas in which pt. is making own decisions & give positive reinforcement to self-enhancing ones; assist with decision-making when profoundly depressed; as depression lifts, expect pt. to make own decisions with support.

Discharge Planning and Teaching Objectives/Outcomes
1) (Patient/Family/Significant Other) Can identify events/loss that led to feeling depressed.
2) Can recall the positive and negative aspects associated with the loss.
3) Can verbally express usual coping mechanisms for dealing with loss and how situational supports can assist to prevent depression.

Recommended References
"Dealing with Depression After Radical Surgery." *Nursing '79*, February 1979:47–49.
"Mr. Jarrett Was Ready to Give Up . . . but I Wasn't," by Diane Cole. *Nursing '78*, March 1978:40–41.
"Programmed Instruction: Helping Depressed Patients in General Nursing Practice." *American Journal of Nursing*, June, 1977:1007–1040.
"Responses to Loss: The Grief and Mourning Process." *NCP Guide* #1:47, 2nd Ed., Nurseco, 1980.
Suicide Assessment and Intervention, by Corrine Hatton et al. New York: Appleton-Century-Crofts, 1977.
"The Patient Experiencing Depression (Psychiatric)." *NCP Guide* #3:35, Nurseco, 1977.
"The Patient Who Is Suicidal." *NCP Guide* #3:38, Nurseco, 1977.

© Margo Creighton Neal, 1980

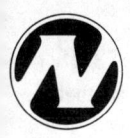

The Patient Experiencing Depression (Psychiatric)

NCP Guide No. **3:35**

Definition: Depression is an affective disorder characterized by an alteration in mood in the direction of abnormally low spirits, and accompanied by intense and sustained feelings of despondence, hopelessness and emptiness.

LONG TERM GOAL: The patient will deal with painful feelings by learning to share, express and resolve them; the patient will resume effective management of own life, as evidenced by ability to carry out activities of daily living and resume job or usual roles.

General Considerations:
- Depression <u>originates</u> as a response to failure or loss. The word "depression" if often used to refer to "the blues" or the sadness and grief that are normal psychological responses to a loss; true depression, however, differs from "the blues" et al, in that the latter are time-limited and proportionate to what was lost. (See NCP Guide #1:31, "Responses to Loss: The Grief and Mourning Process.")
- There are many <u>views and kinds</u> of depression. It may be viewed as (1) <u>a mood state</u> in which the person experiences intense feelings of despair, worthlessness, gloom, emptiness, numbness and a sense of foreboding; as (2) <u>a syndrome or symptom complex</u>: classifications within this category include agitated or retarded depression (refers to motor activity), neurotic or psychotic depression, and reactive or endogenous depression; as (3) <u>a disease process,</u> which includes manic-depressive psychosis, plus involutional, neurotic and psychotic depression; and as (4) <u>a complex of psychodynamic mechanisms:</u> (according to psychoanalytic theory) which views depression as a person's emotional expression of hopelessness and helplessness, characterized by loss of self-esteem in reaction to threatened aspirations and wishes to be loved, worthy and appreciated; to be good, loving and unaggressive; and to be strong, superior and secure.
- <u>Neurotic and psychotic depression</u> have many similarities as well as some marked differences:

	Neurotic	Psychotic
Definition:	A state of depression in which <u>reality testing</u> is largely intact and <u>physiological disturbances,</u> if present, are mild.	A state of depression of psychotic intensity in which <u>reality testing is severely impaired,</u> and <u>physiological</u> disturbances (vegetative signs) <u>are present.</u>
Behaviors:	Sadness, melancholia, crying, withdrawal, difficulty in concentrating, anorexia, slowness of speech and movement, apathetic, little initiative, feels sorry for self, some insight, overt anxiety; behaviors are more severe and last longer than	Marked sadness, extreme melancholia, persistent withdrawal, unable to concentrate, vegetative signs (anorexia, weight loss, constipation, insomnia, AM-PM variations of mood, amenorrhea or impotency), extreme reduction of

with "the blues" or normal reaction to a loss.

physical activity, may be mute or unresponsive, apathetic, no initiative, full of despair: feels everything is coming to an end, little insight, postural muscles seem to sag. Delusions, illusions and hallucinations are rare, but may occur.

Etiology: Loss, failure, guilt, low self-esteem, inability to handle anger (turns toward self, instead of outward to appropriate target). Pre-morbid personality usually contains a milder degree of low self-esteem than in psychotic depression, with a less harsh and punitive superego, less severe feelings of guilt and worthlessness, and more realistic perceptions.

Same as neurotic depression. Pre-morbid personality usually includes chronic low self-esteem, ambivalent feelings about self with harsh & punitive superego leading to feelings of guilt and depreciation of self, unrealistic perceptions of events, feelings. Closely linked with difficulty in interpersonal relations.

- Reactive and Endogenous depressions:

Reactive (or Exogenous)
Precipitating Event: Identifiable.
Behaviors: Responds to environmental stimuli; weight loss less than 10 lbs; feels worse as day progresses; difficulty going to sleep, apathetic.

Etiology: Sudden onset, related to a loss.

Endogenous (aka physiological depression)
Not evident or clear cut.

Does not respond to environmental stimuli; weight loss more than 10 lbs.; feels worse in AM & better as day progresses; may sleep most of day; often awake at 4 or 5 AM; severely retarded thought & actions; responds to meds. & ECT

Onset 1-4 weeks, seems to come from nowhere; tends to be time-limited; possible biochemical aspect; person may have history of family members with depression.

- <u>Treatment</u>: Since there is no right or wrong way to view or define depression, there is no single way to treat it. Somatic therapies of meds. and/or ECT, plus some form of psychotherapy (short-term, crisis intervention, group or family therapy) are generally implemented. (See NCP Guide #3:46, "Drugs: Psychotropic" and #3:47, "Drugs: Tranquilizers.")
- <u>Nursing Responsibilities</u> include assessing the pt's. symptom cluster, helping him to deal with painful feelings, assessing response to somatic therapies, providing support and doing anticipatory planning to prevent and/or cope with future episodes.

Specific Considerations, Potential Patient Outcomes and Nursing Actions:

1) Inability to Cope with Painful Feelings (e.g.   The patient will demonstrate increased ability to cope with painful feelings by accepting nurse's presence, sharing feelings with nurse and others, tolerating experiencing the feelings, exploring ways to cope with the feelings, tolerating reciprocal sharing of feelings with others and resolving the feelings:

The Patient Experiencing Depression (Psychiatric)

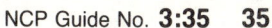

NCP Guide No. **3:35** 35

Sadness, Grief, Guilt, Anger)

- build rapport and relationship with pt. by spending time with him at least twice daily; start with 5-10 mins., and increase time as you and pt. can tolerate it; encourage pt. to identify & share feelings with you, accepting what he says; use silence; just the presence of a caring person is helpful when one is learning to cope with painful feelings; <u>avoid</u> reassurance;
- focus on pt's. feelings; allow him to ventilate in ways that seem comfortable to him; share with pt. that the only to get through feelings is to stay with them & experience them;
- help pt. explore ways to cope with feelings; talk about alternate ways to express them, e.g. to express anger: try handball, racket ball, hitting a punching bag or bed, shouting, singing, confronting with words, swearing, batacus, tearing up phone books, throwing sponges or bean bags. To express guilt: explore situation & persons with whom the pt. experiences guilt: "I feel guilty when I..." Then have pt. try to replace the word "guilt" with "resentment;" explore feelings about this; most situations which involve guilt also involve feelings of anger and resentment; work on these feelings with pt.;
- explore with pt. the persons in his life with whom he is willing to share feelings; if there is no one, explore with him how this came about and his feelings about this situation; if he expresses dissatisfaction with having no one to share feelings with, explore with him ways to change situations; practice using role-playing or psychodrama to try alternative ways to initiate sharing of feelings;
- explore with pt. how he feels about listening to others' feelings; often people who have problems tolerating their own feelings tend to feel overwhelmed with others' feelings; practice sharing feelings of being overwhelmed and setting limits on listening to problems; if other pts. are willing & available, practice reciprocal sharing of feelings, with discussion of how to set limits & keep relationship;
- listen to pt.: focus on meaning of loss, somatic symptoms, feelings tone... "It seems like it just isn't worth it..."; "You've had a hard time lately and you're learning to deal with your feelings;" "You've lost someone you loved and you're going through grief and mourning;" "Sounds like you remember the good parts and the rough parts of this relationship, and you're beginning to be ready to risk again."
- give positive reinforcement to reality and realistic expectations.

2) Inability to Perform Self-Care Activities

Patient will resume self-care in grooming, ingesting adequate foods and fluids, achieving an adequate sleep-rest-activity pattern:
- assess activities of daily living and vegetative signs;

- identify problem areas and work out alternatives with pt. & health team; take care to consider individual preferences & needs; help pt. do things for self (many depressed pts. become dependent on others, but activity usually helps them to feel better);
- assess areas in which pt. is making own decisions and give positive reinforcement to self-enhancing ones; assist with decision-making when profoundly depressed; as depression lifts, expect pt. to make own decisions with support.
- weigh weekly (continued loss of weight may indicate deepened depression; weight gain may indicate decreased depression).
- work with pt. to plan activities of daily living in areas of:
  1) <u>personal appearance</u>: help pt. establish routine for bathing, care of hair, skin, nails, clothes; give positive reinforcement to any care of self;
  2) <u>food intake</u>: work with pt. to find acceptable eating pattern; if pt. is anorexic & apathetic to food, find out when this lessens; could you leave a thermos of hot chocolate, oatmeal cookies, crackers & cheese, 7-Up, etc. at bedside for small snacks at night or day?;
  3) <u>observe sleeping habits:</u> help pt. establish a bedtime routine to promote rest & sleep; without enough sleep, exhaustion may occur & the mental state deteriorate; some depressed people seem to sleep continuously during the day and do not rest at night; work with pt. to mobilize self during day so will be able to rest at night;
  4) plan <u>work assignment</u> with pt.; (daily responsibility for ward maintenance tasks help to renew a sense of self-worth and purposefulness); simple tasks, such as emptying ashtrays, straightening chairs, putting away cards, games or crafts equipment with supervision may be appropriate for deeply depressed pts.; more difficult tasks can be gradually assigned as pt. tolerates;
  5) assess <u>previous hobbies & pastimes</u> which pt. enjoyed; (often depressed persons have few hobbies & haven't participated in recreational or crafts groups since schooldays); simple crafts which can be finished in one sitting give the pt. a therapeutic sense of accomplishment; group singing, poetry reading, painting, working with clay should be encouraged to assist pt. to become more comfortable in groups & establish community & group socialization; pt. may need nurse's presence to tolerate group activities at first; simple exercises, walks, may progress to group sports;
  6) assess <u>bowel habits</u> & work with pt. to choose roughage foods & sufficient fluids if constipated (often resumption of exercise & previous eating habits solves a constipation problem);
  7) assess <u>pt's. knowledge of AM-PM variations in mood</u> & depression; for pts. with endogenous depression, health teach that most pts. feel low in AM & better as the day progresses, especially if they mobilize themselves into activity; for pts. with reactive depression, health teach that their fatigue level affects their depression, so that as day progresses, they may become tired & feel more depressed; if so, they may need to rest in middle of day & do group work in AM, when they feel less depressed;
- if pt. is agitated, above nursing actions may help to rechannel his energy.

The Patient Experiencing Depression (Psychiatric)

NCP Guide No. 3:35

3) Self-Defeating/Destructive Impulses (Related to Overwhelming Feelings of Low Self-esteem, Hopelessness & Helplessness)

Patient will demonstrate increased ability to control self-destructive impulses:
- assess pt.'s impulse control by restricting pt. to observable areas when first admitted; ask pt. if he has thought of hurting himself or suicide (see NCPG #3:38, "Suicide"):
- remove potentially harmful items such as razor blades, scissors & meds., etc. on admission; sharp instruments can be used only with 1-to-1 supervision;
- establish a 1-to-1 relationship with pt.; assess potential for self-defeating acts; problem solve with pt. for alternative behaviors; use role-playing & psychodrama to practice new behaviors;
- work out plan for pt. to use when he feels that he is losing control of his impulses, e.g., contract with pt. that he will ask nurse to accompany him to exercise room so he can hit punching bag when angry at self or others; or contract to spend time with pt. when he experiences increased anxiety or depression, so that he can talk about feelings, cry, rage and not be alone;
- give positive reinforcement by words and nurse's presence when pt. follows through on contract to control impulses... "You really were aware that you were losing control and took good care of yourself by asking me to stay with you."
- retain hope and share it with pt. "I know you are feeling low now; you're getting treatment and these feelings will lift."

4) Social Relationships

Patient will strengthen ability to relate to others by increasing social interactions with staff and other patients:
- assess interpersonal behaviors & help pt. define problem areas in social relationships, e.g., pt. who is hypercritical of self & others can discuss & practice a softer, more accepting approach;
- help pt. to look at situations where he may push people away out of fear of rejection—(reject them before they reject him);
- practice social skills, use role-playing; give positive reinforcement.

Discharge Planning and Teaching Objectives/Outcomes:
1) (Patient and/or family/significant other) Is able to verbalize painful feelings he was experiencing on admission and can contrast them to those he is feeling now.
2) Has a realistic plan for self-care in activities of daily living, as well as for resuming usual job, home or school roles.
3) Has a plan for follow-up care, e.g., Dr., nurse, mental health clinic, etc.

4) Has a written list of medications, schedule and potential side effects; knows where and how to obtain refills and can state importance of taking medications as prescribed.

Recommended References

"Communicating with Depressed Persons," by A. Swanson, <u>Perspectives in Psychiatric Care,</u> April/June, 1975: 63-67.

"The Crying Patient," by Lisa Robinson, <u>Nursing '72</u>, December, 1972: 16-20.

"Depression," by W. Crary & G. Creary, <u>American Journal of Nursing</u>, March, 1973: 472-475.

"Depression: Adaptation to Disruption and Loss," by R. Drake & J. Price, <u>Perspectives in Psychiatric Care,</u> October/December, 1975: 163-169.

"Drugs: Psychotropic," NCP Guide No. 3:46.

"Drugs: Tranquilizers, NCP Guide No. 3:47.

"Intervention in a Schizoaffective Depressive Behavior Pattern: A Behavioral Approach, by J. Provost, <u>Perspectives in Psychiatric Care</u>, April/June, 1974: 86-89.

<u>Psychiatric Nursing in the Hospital and the Community</u>, Ann W. Burgess & A. Lazare, Prentice-Hall, Inc., Englewood Cliffs, N.J., 1976.

"The Patient Who Is Suicidal," NCP Guide No. 3:38.

"Responses to Loss: The Grief and Mourning Process," NCP Guide No. 1:31, NURSECO: 1974.

© Margo Creighton Neal, 1977

NCP Guide No. **4:37** 39

The Patient with a <u>Developmental Disability</u>: <u>Mental Retardation</u> (in an <u>Acute</u> Setting)

LONG TERM GOAL: The patient will maintain admission levels of functioning within limitations imposed by current illness.

General Considerations:
- Read NCPG #4:38, "The Client with a Developmental Disability: Mental Retardation (in a Residential Setting)."
- <u>Incidence</u> of disease/accidents: Retarded persons get their share of acute and chronic diseases and accidents. Certain handicaps are often associated with MR, such as cerebral palsy and epilepsy. An HEW study in 1971 showed that nearly 88% of MR people have at least one additional handicap.
- <u>Nursing responsibilities</u>: respect and consider the retarded person's life experience, years lived, IQ and mental age. Assess abilities and limitations in activities of daily living, social skills, knowledge/attitudes about MR, medical diagnosis and regimen with both patient and family/guardian/significant other (SO). Provide information about regional and national MR organizations as needed and wanted. Provide care dictated by medical diagnosis and regimen, and adapted to accommodate this patient's particular needs and abilities.

Specific Considerations, Potential Patient Outcomes and Nursing Actions:

1) Activities of Daily Living

The patient will maintain admission levels of functioning (state them) in ADL:
- assess pt.'s usual level of ADL by asking pt. and/or family/SO, & adapt these to hospital routine PRN; it is desirable to maintain former patterns & habits to minimize pt.'s anxiety during this period of acute illness or trauma;
- be aware that some regression may occur due to taking on sick role during acute or chronic illness; minimize this by encouraging self-care & work with pt. & family to maintain good health habits & self-care patterns;
- <u>dressing</u>: encourage pt. to dress self in own clothing; if must use hospital clothing, some minor adjustments may help pt. to be independent; allow ample time for dressing & praise positive behaviors;
- <u>bathing and cleaning teeth:</u> help pt. set up convenient routine, using equipment used at home such as electric toothbrush, hairdryer; tactfully observe for cleanliness & assist only if necessary;
- <u>toilet procedures</u>: follow procedure used at home, using usual words & time schedule; may need to remind Q2H or get up at night; do not diaper;
- <u>nutrition</u>: assist pt. to choose foods s/he likes & can manage on diet as ordered; encourage self-help & health-teach to attain understanding of well balanced diet, using simple terms, demonstration & return demonstration of basic food groups, etc.; provide snacks;
- <u>sleep/rest</u>: explain hospital routine & assist pt. to relax during rest periods & sleep at night by following usual sleep routine with

lights, snacks, favored objects, music, etc.

2) Teaching/ Learning Needs	Patient will be able to state/demonstrate (information/procedure) by (set a completion date):

- MR persons often have difficulty with verbal expression & vocabulary, thus behavior modification techniques are effective in learning new tasks, as little verbal exchange is required;
- use pt's own words or teach simple words/concepts; break concept/procedure into small components & allow pt. to practice/talk about each component, giving positive reinforcement & constructive feedback with each practice;
- know that MR persons are easily distracted, thus reducing their ability to concentrate on a specific task; this may lead to feelings of anger, frustration, with subsequent self-injurious behavior such as slapping, biting, banging of head, etc.;
- be creative in adapting pt's. life experience to learning experience;
- health teach family/SO as necessary;
- see NCPGs #1:50, "Teaching Patients: Specific Plan for Skills & Procedures;" #3:32, "Teaching the Parent, Guardian, Child;" and #4:38, "The Client with Mental Retardation (in a Residential Setting)."

3) Medications & Treatments

The patient will accept and show understanding of reasons for medications and treatments by explaining them to nurse in own words:
- prepare pt. for procedures & treatments by explaining ahead of time what to expect & when to expect it, using words pt. understands & asking pt. to repeat what s/he understands in own words;
- listen & learn what pt. expects & help correct misunderstandings;
- maintain uniformity in treatments/procedures & explain changes;
- give emotional support by staying with pt. during treatments/procedures;
- explain to pt. & family necessary information about each medication (name, dosage, time of administration, toxic effects to report); observe & chart observations; spot-check pt's. retention of information; health teaching should be simple, short & relaxed.

4) Safety

The patient will comply with hospital safety rules and will ask for help when s/he needs it:
- explain hospital routine and do's & dont's in simple, relaxed way, including use of call lights, siderails, O_2 or other equipment as necessary; have pt. repeat in own words to facilitate understanding; encourage to ask for help when needed; answer call light promptly;
- assess need for & provide safety devices PRN: e.g. siderails, wheelchair, walker, etc.;
- be aware that many MR pts. tend to put things in their mouth, or do unpredictable things with loose objects; close supervision may be necessary.

The Patient with a <u>Developmental Disability</u>: <u>Mental Retardation</u> (in an <u>Acute</u> Setting)

NCP Guide No. **4:37** 41

5) Psychosocial Adjustment The patient will adapt to hospital setting and will develop and maintain feelings of self-worth:
- respect & consider the pt's. life experience & age regardless of IQ or retardation levels; do not treat the adult person as a child even though his developmental age is that of a child;
- give positive reinforcement to self-help behaviors & socially acceptable attitudes & behaviors; praise healthy habits & attitudes;
- facilitate expression of feelings & encourage pt. to share experience of hospital with nursing staff;
- encourage questions; assign permanent staff to pt. if possible to build trust & rapport;
- spend time & give support to family/guardian/SO; be attentive to information on ADL & health habits; health-teach as necessary; discuss knowledge of regional & national MR services & provide addresses PRN;
- be aware that pt. & SO/family/guardian/caretaker may have unusual degree of emotional dependence due to limitations of retarded person in daily life.

Discharge Planning and Teaching Objectives/Outcomes:
1) (Patient/Family/Guardian) Has received and can verbalize understanding of written set of instructions re: medications, diet, exercise, treatments.
2) Verbalizes knowledge of all prescribed medications with name, dosage, administration times and directions, side effects.
3) Has information/appointment for next contact with physician.
4) Expresses knowledge of regional or national center for MR and has address(es) to contact them for services.
5) Has been evaluated for assistance (financial, vocational, home health care) and appropriate referral made.
6) Is aware that hospital/clinic is willing to collaborate with community agencies for reports, future care.

Recommended References
"Behavior Modification by Parents in Home," by B. Haus et al, <u>Journal of Psychiatric Nursing</u>, August 1976: 9-16.
"The Client with a Developmental Disability: Mental Retardation (in a Residential Setting)," <u>NCP Guide</u>, #4:38, Nurseco, 1978.
"No Pity," by B. Barbieri, <u>American Journal of Nursing</u>, September 1976: 1482.
"OR Nursing Care for the Retarded," by S. Roy, <u>AORN</u>, October 1976: 672-678.
"Preparation of Mental Health Personnel for the Delivery of Mentally Retarded Services," by A. Hersh et al, <u>Journal of Community Mental Health</u>, September 1977: 13-23.
"Teaching Patients: Specific Plan for Skills and Procedures," <u>NCP Guides</u> #1:50, Nurseco, 1974.
"Teaching the Parent/Guardian/Child: General Suggestions," <u>NCP Guides</u> #3:32, Nurseco, 1977.
"Understanding & Helping the Mentally Retarded," by G. Dodge, <u>AORN</u>, October 1976: 679-684.

The Client with a <u>Developmental Disability</u>: <u>Mental Retardation</u> (in a <u>Residential</u> Setting)

NCP Guide No. **4:38**

Definition: Mental retardation (MR) as defined by the American Association on Mental Deficiency refers to a sub-average general intellectual functioning which originates during the developmental period and is associated with impairment in adaptive behavior.

LONG TERM GOAL: The resident will learn to perform self-care activities with maximum independence for developmental level; will develop and maintain feelings of self-worth.

General Considerations:
- <u>Manifestations</u> of MR include: poor learning, inadequate social adjustment, and delayed or lowered potential capacity for achievement.
- <u>Causes</u>:
    <u>Before birth</u>: genetic variations (Down's syndrome or mongolism, Tay-Sachs), German measles or infection in mother during pregnancy, incompatible blood between mother and child (RH factor), glandular disorders, toxic chemicals.
    <u>During birth</u>: birth injury due to long and difficult labor or very rapid delivery, abnormal position of fetus, difficult forceps delivery.
    <u>After birth</u>: inflammation of the brain from high fever due to childhood diseases, accident with trauma to head; glandular disturbances, inadequate stimulation in early childhood.
- <u>Levels</u> of retardation (Classification system of American Association of Mental Deficiency):
    <u>Borderline</u> (Level 0)—IQ range 68 to 83, with a potential adult mental age (MA) level of 10 years, 11 months to 13 years, 3 months; usually capable of marriage and being self-supporting, probably at a low socio-economic living standard.
    <u>Mild or educable</u> (Level 1)—IQ range 52 to 67, with a potential adult MA level of 8 years, 6 months to 10 years, 10 months; capable of working but needs some supervision in financial affairs. Fourth/fifth grade academic possibilities as well as vocational skills by adulthood; often has difficulty keeping a job in competitive market. School placement is usually in classes for the educable mentally retarded (EMR); can usually be maintained within a community setting.
    <u>Moderate</u> (Level 2)—IQ range 36 to 51, with a potential adult MA level of 6 years, 1 month to 8 years, 5 months; first to third grade academic potential. Vocational possibilities usually at sheltered workshop or neighborhood job; school placement is usually in classes for trainable mentally retarded (TMR).
    <u>Severe</u> (Level 3)—IQ range 20 to 35, with a potential adult MA level of 3 years, 9 months to 6 years; training goals are largely the self-help skills (toilet training, dressing self), with minimal independent behavior; school placement is usually in a developmental center for handicapped or TMR

program; some are able to work in sheltered workshop.

    Profound (Level 4)—IQ below 20, and adult MA potential is 3 to 8 years and below; often accompanied by damage to CNS. Person may require total care.

- **Incidence:** estimated 6 million MR individuals in U.S. in 1976; one out of 10 American families has an MR member; 70-80% are in the borderline or mild (EMR) category; <u>20-30% are moderately, severely or profoundly retarded. The latter are most often cared for in residential institutions.</u>
- **Factors** found to promote residential self-sufficiency, adjustment and mental growth include: (1) clinical staff giving individual attention via affection, conversation, meeting physical needs; (2) residents having less contacts with MR peers and aides and more contact with non-MR persons and professional staff; and (3) staffing tends to small groups with primary staff consistently responsible for same residents.
- **Treatment:** Although the intelligence of the MR usually cannot be increased, much can be done to teach and reinforce socially desirable behaviors and attitudes, self-care activities of daily living, and to increase the quality of life.
- **Nursing responsibilities:** include showing respect and consideration of resident's experience and years lived, as well as IQ & MA; working with interdisciplinary team to assess resident's needs, to plan and evaluate an individual program to help resident function at optimum level; observing & reporting physical signs & symptoms which might indicate a communicable disease, infection, etc.; helping resident and/or family prepare for future via health teaching and possible return to home or community placement.

Specific Considerations, Potential Patient Outcomes and Nursing Actions:

1) Activities of Daily Living (ADL)

The resident will perform self-care in hygiene and grooming (and other ADL as appropriate for individual):
- assess ability to perform ADL including toileting, bathing, brushing teeth & hair, shampooing, shaving, nail care, dressing;
- identify areas of learning needs & teach activities to meet those needs.

2) Teaching/ Learning Needs

The resident will learn (state specific) skill/procedure by (set a completion date):
- assess learning needs & health teach in areas of self-care, family life, sex education, family planning & VD counseling;
- know that MR residents tend to have decreased verbal skills & comprehension, and that problems with attention span are acute in the severely & profoundly MR groups; use few words & more demonstration, for short periods of time;
- choose a priority from the learning needs and focus on only one activity, skill or procedure at a time; choose time of day when resident is rested & alert; choose an appropriate teaching area with minimal distractions;
- write out the exact steps of the skill the resident is to learn: break down to the most elemental components; arrange the steps in logical sequence (this is called <u>chaining</u>); always teach the chain in this <u>exact</u> order; use <u>backwards chaining with MR</u>, i.e. <u>teach last step first</u> and work backwards through entire procedure, e.g. <u>13 steps to wash & dry hands:</u>

    1. dispose of paper towel in container   2. dry hands
    3. take paper towel   4. remove plug from sink

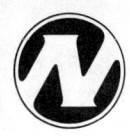

The Client with a <u>Developmental Disability</u>: <u>Mental Retardation</u> (in a <u>Residential</u> Setting)

    5. rinse soap from hands   6. scrub hands
    7. put soap on hands   8. wet hands
    9. place water in sink   10. place plug in sink
   11. turn off cold water   12. turn on cold water
   13. point to cold water tap on command

- teach only 1 or 2 steps of the chain in one session, or as you assess the resident can comprehend;
- guide, assist or "walk" person through the actual procedure PRN, e.g. hold their hand while turning on faucet, or picking up food with a spoon;
- urge resident to practice & reward any behavior that comes close to desired behavior;
- increase learning with use of praise & rewards that are important to resident, e.g. desired privileges, time with a friend or staff, music, TV, sugar-free gum, extra time out of doors; use food or candy as last resort as they tend to lead to overweight and dental caries;
- respond immediately if resident stops attending to lesson: say "no," and ignore for 15 sec., then resume teaching;
- bring reward/reinforcer to learner's attention PRN, e.g. hold gum at eye level and when learner attends, show next step & give him the gum after s/he performs the step;
- reward ever-longer chains (larger # of steps) until entire sequence is learned, then reward only completion of total task; have resident practice in different settings to promote transfer of behavior;
- be consistent, positive & patient;
- when one skill is learned completely & adequately for that individual, repeat process with next skill or learning need.

3) Rest & Exercise

<u>The ambulatory resident</u> will preserve and improve independent functioning such as range of motion, strength, tolerance, coordination:
- work with PT & OT staff to assess, plan, implement & evaluate an activity/exercise program to meet resident's needs;
- record kind & amount of exercise & ability to do same, as well as resident's reactions, tolerance & coordination in ADL.

<u>The multiple-handicapped & non-ambulatory resident</u> will spend a major portion of waking hours out of bed, out of bedroom area, with some time out of doors daily; will have planned daily activity & exercise periods; will experience mobility and self-care whenever possible:

- work with interdisciplinary team to assess, plan & implement daily activity/exercise schedule for resident; provide ROM or other exercise PRN; help resident to participate in group activities;
- observe resident's reactions to group activities; give positive reinforcement for positive behaviors, i.e. cooperation, support of other residents, enthusiasm, initiating interactions; work with resident to develop individual free time recreational activities;
- encourage resident to work with & take care of own personal possessions such as games, arts & crafts materials, books, radios;
- refer to NCPG #2:45, "Hazards of Immobility, and NCPG #1:47, "Range of Motion Exercises."

4) Nutrition   The resident will ingest adequate food and fluids and will eat in a manner consistent with developmental needs:
- supervise meal times PRN to ensure resident ingests an adequate amount of food; help resident to eat sitting at table in dining room, assessing areas where teaching is needed;
- give positive reinforcement to positive eating skills;
- use adaptive equipment PRN; chain components as in 2) above;
- chart intake with % of meal eaten.

5) Medications & Treatments   The resident will ingest prescribed medications in a safe manner:
- when giving oral meds. ensure that resident swallows them;
- observe for adverse effects of meds. & report any immediately;
- health-teach effects of meds. and self-administration as appropriate for MA;
- know that there seems to be a greater incidence of allergic reactions to drugs, food, and other substances among the MR;
- many people with MR have one or more handicaps and may need ongoing treatments; acquaint yourself with Rx. procedures, explaining each step to resident.

6) Psychosocial Adjustment   The resident will develop/maintain feelings of self-worth:
- respect & consider the resident's life experience & age regardless of his IQ or MA levels; treat as an adult, even though his developmental age may be that of a child;
- provide opportunities to spend time with a staff person or do small tasks, such as errands, etc.;
- give praise for efforts to maintain grooming, carry out ADL; give recognition to a new pair of shoes, haircut, dress, etc.;
- provide choices for resident, so that s/he has options, rather than a "you must do this now";
- consider individual limitations & disabilities & find some things for resident to do at which he can achieve some degree of success;
- help resident vent anger & sort out the problem that caused it; frustration & anger often appear in MR residents due to poor verbal & communication skills; much patience may be needed to understand what resident is feeling;

NCP Guide No. **4:38** 47

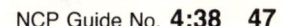

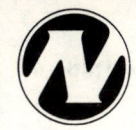

The Client with a <u>Developmental Disability</u>: <u>Mental Retardation</u> (in a <u>Residential</u> Setting)

- distract pt. from potentially violent behavior into another activity; refer to NCPG #4:40, "The Violent Patient";
- work with social worker & other staff to help resident's family develop constructive & personally meaningful ways to support resident's experience in the institution;
- work with family to prepare for resident's return home or community placement.

Discharge Planning and Teaching Objectives/Outcomes:
See this Section in NCPG #4:37, "The Patient with a Developmental Disability: Mental Retardation (in an Acute Setting)."
1) If a home or community placement is possible, (the resident) can carry out self-care activities (state them).

Recommended References
"The Agonizing Decisions in Mental Retardation," Rosalee C. Yeaworth, <u>American Journal of Nursing</u>, May 1977: 864-867.
"Behavior Modification and Therapy in Mental Retardation," by N. Hyde, <u>American Journal of Nursing</u>, May 1974: 883-886.
"Hazards of Immobility," <u>NCP Guide</u> #2:45, Nurseco, 1975.
<u>The Mentally Retarded: Answers to Questions About Sex</u>, by A. Attwell & C. Jamison, Western Psychological Services, Los Angeles: 1977 (an excellent reference for sexuality, VD, family counseling for MR).
<u>Mental Retardation: Nature, Cause and Management</u>, by G. Baroff, New York: Wiley & Sons, 1974.
"Nurses Can Be Effective Behavior Modifiers," by Y.D. Neimeier and T. Allison, <u>Journal of Psychiatric Nursing and Mental Health Services</u>, January 1976: 18-21.
"Range of Motion Exercises," <u>NCP Guide</u> #1:47, Nurseco, 1974.
"Where Hope for Mental Retardees Grows Brighter," by I. Horoshak, <u>RN</u>, June 1976: 39-43.

© Margo Creighton Neal, 1978

NCP Guide No. 4:38 48

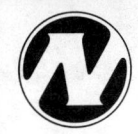

The Patient Experiencing Fear

Definition: An emotional response to a consciously recognized internal and/or external source of danger.

LONG TERM GOAL: The patient will be able to interact with the environment in such a way that s/he recognizes factors and situations that cause him to be fearful.

General Considerations:
— **Fear** is a response that occurs in all individuals but can become especially acute in those with no previous hospitalization or with a previous traumatic experience. Fear may also present itself when a person associates his own anticipated experience with the traumatic experience of another, eg. family member, friend, job associate.
— **Nursing assessment** includes observing for behavioral manifestations of fear which include:
- refusal of treatment;
- putting on call light frequently;
- making constant, unnecessary demands on staff;
- constant attempts to please staff and do "what's right";
- constant crying;
- aggressive and/or critical with staff;
- feeling a sinking sensation in stomach;
- somatic complaints, such as nausea, diarrhea;
- constant questioning about a care activity;
- increased vital signs, perspiration.

It also includes the assessment of the patient's response to the diagnosis, treatment and/or hospitalization in order to determine those activities or events which have caused the fear. It may be necessary to explore the intrapsychic meaning of the event(s) and relationship to a previous experience in order to determine the root of the fear.
— **Nursing responsibilities** include assessment and intervention which focuses on eliminating or reducing to a minimum the source of the fear, while enhancing the patient's control over other aspects of his care. Remember that loss of structure or loss of flexibility in daily living style can increase the intensity of the fear.

Specific Considerations, Potential Patient Outcomes, and Nursing Actions:

1) Immediate Response to Recognition of Fear

The patient will be able to identify the fear and its cause:
— attempt to identify the specific source of the fear;
— use indirect, open-ended questions such as, "What is it about being in the hospital that concerns you most?"
— give careful explanation of all that is to occur to the pt.; following explanations, have pt. tell you in his own words what you said & what it means to him; repeat this procedure as often as needed to ensure the pt.'s understanding;
— if you are unable to reduce the fear (eg. of dying during surgery) prior to the event, notify Dr. so appropriate corrective action can be taken; surgery may be cancelled.

2) Restoration to Adaptive Coping

The patient will be able to discuss his fears with others and accept treatment:
— spend at least 15 mins. with pt. each day; direct the conversation towards his responses to the hospital: "What thoughts are you having about the way your hospitalization is going?"
— listen to & positively reinforce the pt.'s attempt to talk about decisions that involve dangerous procedures or major life changes;
— do not make the decisions for the pt.;
— verbally & non-verbally assist the pt. in asking questions s/he may have about the progress and/or outcome of his diagnosis & treatment;
— direct questions about diagnosis & treatment not appropriate to nursing to the physician & explain the reason the pt. needs the answer, e.g. he is afraid of the outcome of his illness;
— involve & give explanation to other interested persons so they may reinforce the teaching you have done;
— allow friends & family to express their fears so they will be comfortable & supportive to the pt.; this intervention will be important in preventing the pt. from the realization of a fear of abandonment.

Discharge Planning and Teaching Objectives/Outcomes

1) (Patient/Family/Significant Other) Can verbally identify those aspects of own body and health care that cause fear.
2) Can utilize situational supports to reduce fear and accept treatment.
3) Can discuss information about developments in health care to prevent unwarranted fears.

Recommended References

"A Better Way to Calm the Patient Who Fears the Worst." *RN*. April 1977:46–33.
"Gaining Insight into Fear." *Nursing '78*, April 1978:46–51.
"Psychological Responses in Critical Care Units," by Margaret Adams et al. *American Journal of Nursing*, September 1978:1504–1512.
"The Frightened Patient," by Lisa Robinson. *Psychological Aspects of the Care of Hospitalized Patients*, 2nd ed., Philadelphia: F.A. Davis Co., 1972.

© Margo Creighton Neal, 1980

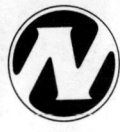

The Patient Experiencing Guilt

Definition: Guilt is a subjective feeling of remorse and self-reproach stemming from a belief that one has done wrong, or has transgressed a social or moral code, or value system.

LONG TERM GOAL: The patient will express and explore guilt feelings and will develop alternative ways of coping with the situation that produced the guilt.

General Considerations:
— Social and moral codes develop early in life from interaction with significant others; cultural, ethnic, religious, and family values are internalized.
— The mature and well-adjusted person can discriminate between current adult situations and past childhood situations to update and affirm values.
— **Behavioral manifestations** and feelings of guilt may include:
  - feelings of remorse or regret;
  - feelings of disgrace and dishonor;
  - expectation of reproach from significant others;
  - self-punishment;
  - preoccupation with situation;
  - labels self in negative way;
  - inability to forgive self;
  - excessive stress level.
— **Causes** of guilt in a hospital setting may include:
  - patient believes that s/he has actually or potentially injured self or another person by accident or neglect;
  - patient has physically or emotionally abused someone else;
  - patient has given birth or parented child with genetic or birth defect;
  - noncompliance with health care plan.
— Repentance tasks allow the individual to repent or apologize for wrongdoing and be forgiven by significant others, social or religious group. The process of repentance facilitates self-forgiveness.
— The healthy person learns from mistakes and modifies behaviors with integrity to avoid transgressing values and moral codes.

Specific Considerations, Potential Patient Outcomes, and Nursing Actions:

1) Immediate Response to Recognition of Guilt

   The patient will express feelings of guilt, remorse, and self-reproach:
   — observe for excessive stress level; assist pt. to use adaptive coping mechanisms to obtain relief from stress; see NCPG #5:49, "Stress Management;"
   — make frequent intermittent contact with the pt., both verbal & non-verbal to offer support, build rapport and trust relationships;
   — offer self as non-judgmental listener; encourage expression of feelings; reflect & summarize pt's. words, e.g., "You seem to feel as though you could have prevented your stroke. Tell me more about that," or "You wish you hadn't spoken so sharply to your daughter?" or "Sounds like you can't forgive yourself for not going to the doctor when you first found the lump."

2) Identification of Values and Moral Codes

   The patient will identify the moral code or value system transgressed:
   — allow pt. to talk about transgression;
   — encourage pt. to identify moral code or value system s/he has transgressed;
   — identify source of moral code or value in life experience, i.e., family, culture, religion:
   — explore pt.'s present value system;
   — check reality of transgression: was it real or fantasy?
   — support realistic assessment of the situation;
   — explore ways to repent or apologize for real transgression, e.g., is pt. willing to talk about incident with daughter to validate that she perceived her mother as "talking sharply"? Is pt. sorry? Is she willing to tell daughter she is sorry and ask forgiveness? Is she willing to forgive herself? Pt. may repent by being "good pt." and by cooperating with treatment plan, physical therapy, diet, medications, etc.

3) Alternative Coping Methods

   The patient will develop new ways of coping with the transgression:
   — assess for lack of knowledge about defense mechanisms & responses to loss & grief; health teach as needed;
   — assist pt. to identify other persons who may be available to share common problems;
   — encourage pt. to discuss feelings & values with trusted person; help pt. to reach out for emotional support;
   — know that self-forgiveness is an important component of mental health; emphasize the need for realistic expectations for

self & others; see NCPG #5:35, "The Patient Experiencing Shame/Embarrassment" & #5:32, "The Patient Experiencing a Threat to Self-Esteem;"
— discuss & problem solve alternative ways of behaving in situations which produced guilt; explore pros & cons of these new ways, & encourage pt. to anticipate his response to them; see NCPG #5:47, "Problem Solving;"
— observe for continued high stress level or continued unresolved feelings of guilt; refer to chaplain or psychiatric nurse specialist.

Discharge Planning and Teaching Objectives/Outcomes
1) (Patient/Family/Significant Other) Can identify situations in which s/he feels guilty.
2) Has developed alternative ways of adaptively coping with guilt feelings.

Recommended References
"The Effect of Hospitalization on Guilt and Shame Feelings," by Ilhan M. Ermutlu. *Psychiatric Forum*, Winter 1977:18–23.
"Guilt and the Working Mother," by S.L. Rad. *American Baby*, January 1980:54–55.
"The Patient Experiencing Shame/Embarrassment." *NCP Guide #5:35*, Nurseco, 1981.
"The Patient Experiencing a Threat to Self-Esteem." *NCP Guide #5:32*, Nurseco, 1981.
Patient Problems in Self-Esteem and Nursing Intervention, by Merle Mishel. Los Angeles: California State University Press. 1976:52–53, 118.
"Problem Solving." *NCP Guide #5:47*, Nurseco, 1981.
"Shame," by Silvia Lange. *Behavioral Concepts & Nursing Intervention*, Carolyn Carlson & Betty Blackwell, Eds. Philadelphia: J.B. Lippincott Co., 1978:54–71.
"Spiritual Dimensions of Nursing Practice," by Jean Stallwood and Ruth Stoll. *Clinical Nursing*, Irene Beland & Joyce Passos, Eds. New York: Macmillan. 1975:1086–1089.
"Stress Management." *NCP Guide #5:49*, Nurseco, 1981.

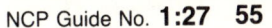

Dealing with Impending Death

NCP Guide No. **1:27** 55

Definition: The process or threat of loss of life.

LONG TERM GOAL: The patient will verbalize an understanding of what is occurring and how s/he is coping with it.

General Considerations:
- **Impending death** can occur as a response to traumatic events, short or long term illness. No matter the source, it causes the patient to bring forth whatever defenses s/he may have available.
- **Working through** the feelings and concerns associated with impending death involves five major stages, according to Kubler-Ross (see Recommended References). This is comparable to the three stages of the grief and mourning process as described in NCPG #1:31.
- **Lack of resolution** of any stage or completion of the total process may be related to the patient's fear of "acceptance" of death, and therefore loss of his ability to "hope" or desire to believe he will not die.
- **Nursing assessment** includes both physical and emotional needs of the patient: *physical needs*—explanations and information desired for decision making about ongoing medical treatment, level of treatment desired by the patient; pain tolerance and how the patient copes with pain, level of pain medication indicated and desired; nutritional preferences; cosmetic needs, including desire for wig, make up, prothesis; general comfort measures needed by the patient, e.g. frequent change of position, timing of procedures, interval of physical care; *emotional needs*—usual method of coping with threats and fears; desire for spiritual assistance; cultural and family practices desired by the patient; desire to talk about impending death with someone who will listen; patient and significant others' beliefs about patient's condition.
- **Nursing responsibilities** include a working knowledge of the grief and mourning process in order to make a nursing diagnosis, knowledge of resources available to the patient and his family, e.g. hospice care, thanotologists (a specialist in care of the dying), bereavement groups for the survivors. Interventions are directed toward comfort and supportive measures that assist the patient to cope *in his own way* with impending death. The only control the patient may feel s/he has at this time is control of how, when and with whom s/he dies. As much as is legally possible, do not take this control away from the patient.

Specific Considerations, Potential Patient Outcomes, and Nursing Actions:

1) Stage I: Denial and Isolation

The patient will be able to use these coping mechanisms to begin to deal with his impending death:
- allow the pt. to utilize own method of coping as long as s/he is not physically destructive;
- know that pt. may have a feeling of "the need to protect others," to "fight the battle alone"; be available to spend at least 10 minutes with him daily either conversing or just being with him;
- assist the pt. to realize that denial and isolation are "normal" reactions to the news of the impending loss of life;

- answer questions about life, death & treatment honestly; the pt. doesn't want you to be harsh in your honesty, but s/he also doesn't want to be "fooled"; leave room in your answers for the pt. to maintain hope if s/he chooses to do so;
- do not reinforce pt.'s denial of his condition; when s/he makes an unrealistic statement ("I'm going to be back to work soon."), respond in a realistic manner, e.g. "It must be difficult for you right now."

2) Stage II: Anger The patient will be able to express anger verbally about his impending death:
- allow & encourage the verbal expression of anger: remember, s/he is thinking, "Why does it have to be me?"; often this feeling is displaced on others; it is not personally directed at you but is a coping strategy that the pt. is using (see "The Patient Manifesting Anger," NCP Guide No. 1:21);
- know that the anger may be self-directed & associated with guilt about not seeking medical attention earlier; allow the pt. to express these concerns but not ruminate on them;
- allow open discussion of alternative treatment & life style options brought up by the pt.; assist him in consideration of these by giving clear, factual information about any alternatives; remember it is the pt.'s choice;
- listen to pt. express anger about distancing behavior from relatives & friends.

3) Stage III: Bargaining The patient will be able to utilize this coping mechanism and associated behavior to try to prolong life;
- allow the pt. to cope by bargaining; s/he may use phrases such as "If only . . ." or "I could do . . .";
- ask the pt. about the importance of the events s/he is bargaining for; in this way, you express your availability to listen to him talk about his feelings;
- part of the bargaining may include the timing & interval of treatment or lack of such; allow the pt. the opportunity to make such decisions; be sure s/he is aware of the risks & consequences but allow him the decision.

4) Stage IV: Depression The patient will verbally recognize the inevitable and allow himself to feel sad;
- know that the pt. may express the sadness verbally or by crying, silence, or talking; when pt. attempts to share sadness, do not try to cheer him up, but acknowledge his feelings;
- such questions as, "Am I going to die?" are a test of staff's willingness to listen to the pt. talk about his concerns, sadness & fears; respond, "Do you feel you are going to die?" then support & discuss responses;
- be aware that during this stage the pt. may be so overwhelmed with sadness that s/he no longer wants to talk or be involved in treatment; s/he may feel, "What difference does it make?"; focus on the normalcy of feeling sad & ascertain with him what difference coping with the impending death rather than giving up, will make to him;
- if pt. chooses not to move beyond this stage, feeling that if s/he stays depressed s/he does not have to make a decision about "fighting or accepting" death, gently remind him that staying depressed involves making a decision not to make another decision.

5) Stage V: Resolution — The patient will accept the impending death as inevitable;
- acceptance involves the realization that death will occur & in preparation for such, the pt. has taken care of personal & family matters; is able to say death will occur & stops his struggle;
- know that often acceptance is not achieved but resignation is the method of resolution; resignation involves realizing that death will occur, but does not want it to happen, struggle continues & the pt. is not at peace with himself;
- spend time with pt.; encourage family & friends to continue to visit; the pt. does not want to be alone;
- the family may not be at the same level of coping as the pt.; share time with them discussing their feelings;
- allow the pt. control; encourage him to direct his care as much as possible; ask him what after death care he would like, i.e. spiritual care, funeral arrangements, family to be called.

Recommended References

"A Philosophy of Death Made Personal," by Sharon Hendrickson. *American Journal of Nursing*, January 1976:90.
"Dare to Care for the Dying," by Joy K. Ifemce. *American Journal of Nursing*, January 1976:88–90.
"Dealing Naturally with Dying," by Robert E. Kavanaugh. *Nursing '76*, October 1976:22–29.
"Experiences with Dying Patients." *American Journal of Nursing*—Feature Series, June 1973:1038.
"Hospice Home Care Program," by Barbara J. Ward. *Nursing Outlook*, October 1978:646–649.
On Death and Dying, by Elizabeth Kubler-Ross. New York: Macmillan Co., 1969.
"Surviving," by Patricia Chaney, Ed. *Nursing '76*, April 1976:41–50.
"The Advanced Cancer Patient: How He Will Live—And Die," by Ruth McCorkle. *Nursing '76*, October 1976:46–49.
"The Fine Example," by Dorothy W. Kimble. *Nursing '76*, July 1976:44.
"To Sharon with Love," by Maureen Cannon. *American Journal of Nursing*, April 1979:642–645.

© Margo Creighton Neal, 1980 **Dealing with Impending Death** NCP Guide No. 1:27.

NCP Guide No. 1:27 58

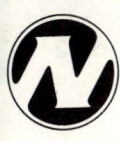

The Patient Experiencing a Threat to Self-Esteem

Definition: **Self-esteem** is the perception or evaluation of oneself based on the quality of relationships with significant others, life experiences, and body image.

Body image is an inner sense of identity which includes body functions, abilities, and limitations.

A **threat** to self-esteem can be any event which negatively alters the individual's perception or evaluation of self.

LONG TERM GOAL: The patient will be able to cope adaptively with a threat to self-esteem and maintain/regain a realistic perception of self.

General Considerations:

— **Common causes** of a threat to self-esteem include:
- loss of significant other due to divorce, death, or disagreement;
- body image disturbance due to real or anticipated loss of body part or function (see NCPG #2:29, "Body Image Disturbance");
- role change, such as change in family or work role, well role to sick role (see NCPG #5:36, "Adapting to Sick Role");
- chronic illness with limitations and lifestyle changes; and
- aging.

— **Common behaviors** of a threat to self-esteem include:
- moderate to high anxiety (see NCPG #1:22, "Anxiety");
- negative labeling of self—example, "I'm just a burden," "I'm only a housewife," "I'm stupid;"
- devaluing of self; feels unliked, unloveable;
- tendency to withdraw by removing self from social situations, avoiding threatening subjects or situations; may be fearful, rigid;
- tendency to submit and be passive, non-assertive, compliant;
- aggressive and hostile behaviors; mistrust;
- feels powerless and unable to see alternatives in situations; and
- use of defense mechanisms such as denial, intellectualization.

— **Nursing responsibilities** include assessing patient for behaviors associated with threat to self-esteem, choosing interventions to facilitate coping with the threat, and providing anticipatory guidance for coping with future threats.

Specific Considerations, Potential Patient Outcomes, and Nursing Actions:

1) Immediate Response to Recognition of Threat to Self-Esteem

The patient will be able to explore feelings, perception of self, and source of threat:
— provide openings for pt. to express feelings by validating your observations (e.g., "You look upset . . . what is happening with you?");
— accept pt.'s feelings & explore further; focus on pt.'s perception of self & events; do not challenge unrealistic perceptions or defensive behaviors;
— listen for & assist pt. to identify the sources of the threats; utilize reality testing to evaluate the perception of the threat (e.g., does pt. have correct information? Does pt. perceive his own abilities accurately? Is there some past experience that makes this situation threatening?); identify & explore distortion of reality;
— validate own knowledge of the components of the threatening situation with health team, pt., physician, chart, & textbooks (e.g., prognosis, treatment, side effects, etc.);
— offer safe, supportive atmosphere of respect & calm attentiveness to pt. needs & concerns; provide for basic needs and activities of daily living (ADL);
— assess anxiety level & facilitate coping with anxiety (see NCPG #1:22);
— assess for knowledge of appropriate behaviors of current health role & health teach as needed (see NCPGs #5:36, "Sick Role" & #5:30, "Chronic Illness Role").

2) Restoration to Adaptive Coping

The patient will explore own strengths and past coping mechanisms; the patient will plan ADL:
— explore past coping mechanisms & abilities; assist pt. to generalize from past, successful coping to present threat situation; focus on strengths & assets;
— allow pt. to make as many decisions as possible in ADL (e.g., planning time of treatments, ambulation, hold visitors/ phone, selecting menu);
— give positive reinforcement, using words & active listening, as pt. explores strengths & makes decisions on ADL;
— involve significant others & family to support pt. in adaptive coping with threat by non-judgmental listening, acceptance, hopeful attitude, & touch;
— assess pt.'s knowledge of relaxation techniques & health teach as needed; encourage diversionary activities, hobbies, exercise as appropriate to pt.'s physical condition.

3) Anticipatory Guidance to Future Threats

The patient will problem solve for alternative options to cope with threat to self-esteem:
— problem solve to explore pros & cons of alternative coping responses (refer to NCPG #5:47, "Problem Solving"); role play to practice alternative behaviors in small units so that the pt. can select most adaptive coping response & experience success;
— explore pt.'s negative expectations with him, focusing on questioning: Why do I have this expectation? Where does it come from? What person in my past (mother, father, friend) would agree with this negative expectation? What purpose does it serve? Does it realistically describe my here-and-now experiences?
— facilitate anticipation of possible future threats; using role playing & behavioral rehearsal, assist pt. to cope effectively in behavioral trial runs;
— reinforce, using words & behavior, realistic, positive anticipation of coping effectively with threat;
— assess learning needs for communications of feelings & ideas, for asking to have needs met; teach communication skills & assertion techniques as needed;
— teach pt. to develop positive affirmations about self, such as "I am flexible and calm," "I am a person who can learn and grow," "I am growing stronger and healthier," "I can learn from difficult relationships and situations."

Discharge Planning and Teaching Objectives/Outcomes

1) (Patient/Family/Significant Other) Can recognize and demonstrate increased ability to cope with threat to self-esteem.
2) Can describe a realistic perception of self.

Recommended References

"Becoming An Assertive Nurse," by D. Bakdash. *American Journal of Nursing*, October 1978:1710–1712.
"Developing a Child's Self-Esteem," by R. Fleming. *Pediatric Nursing*, July–August 1979:58–60.
"The Patient Experiencing a Body Image Disturbance." *NCP Guide #2:29*, 2nd Ed., Nurseco, 1980.
"The Patient Experiencing Anxiety." *NCP Guide #1:22*, 2nd Ed., Nurseco, 1980.
"The Patient Adapting to Chronic Illness Role." *NCP Guide #5:30*, Nurseco, 1981.
"The Patient Adapting to the Sick Role." *NCP Guide #5:36*, Nurseco, 1981.
Patient Problems in Self-Esteem and Nursing Intervention by Merle Mishel. Los Angeles: California State University Press, 1976.
"Problem Solving." *NCP Guide #5:47*, Nurseco, 1981.
"Reminiscence, Self-Esteem and Self-Other Satisfactions in Adult Male Alcoholics," by D. Gibson. *Journal of Psychiatric Nursing*, March 1980:7–11.
"Self-Concept and Mastectomy," by H. Jenkins. *Journal of Geriatric Nursing*, January–February 1980:38–42.
"Supporting the Hospitalized Elderly Patient," by Ann Lore. *American Journal of Nursing*, March 1979:496–499.

NCP Guide No. **3:36** 63

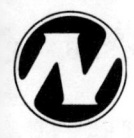

The Patient with <u>Manic-Depressive Psychosis</u>

Definition: Manic-depressive psychosis is an affective disorder characterized by recurring opposite emotional states of mania and depression.

LONG TERM GOAL: The patient will resume effective management of own life, and will be able to identify those behaviors indicative of an approaching manic or depressive episode.

General Considerations:
- The patient <u>manifests</u> intense mood swings of elation or depression, lasting 2-3 months to 2 years, if untreated. The mood swings may be gradual or quite sudden.
- <u>Occurs</u> more often in women than in men, and more often in the upper socio-economic classes. The first clear-cut episodes usually occur in the 30's, but careful history-taking often reveals that there were significant fluctuations in mood at an earlier age. Some patients seem to have an annual or seasonal pattern to their mood swings, while others follow a random course.
- The manic-depressive syndrome is considered to be an <u>endogenous depression</u>; recurrent attacks of mania with or without depression are called <u>bipolar depression</u>; recurrent attacks of depression with no manic attack are called <u>unipolar depression.</u>
- <u>Common behaviors include</u>:
  - <u>manic phase</u>: an affect of euphoria and elation, impulsive behavior, e.g. sudden trips or spending money wildly, no worries, may neglect self; does not have time to eat, sleep, dress; increased verbal and motor activity. May have loose associations with "flight of ideas" (thought sequence characterized by rapid speech, disconnected change of topics; tends to be incomprehensible to listener.)
  - in <u>hypomania</u> (a milder form of mania), patient may eat voraciously, experience increased sexual interest, and go for long periods of time without sleep and without appearing fatigued.
  - in a <u>fully-developed mania</u>, patient may experience delusions, unrealistic ideas of an expansive, grandiose nature, motor activity may increase to a degree that patient cannot focus on food, caring for self, or sexual performance; when this happens, the hyperactivity may become life-threatening as the patient does not eat, drink or sleep; weight loss is common, speech is incoherent, activity is ceaseless and wild, and impulsive, destructive acts towards any person in the environment may occur.
  - <u>depressive phase</u>: see "endogenous depression," in NCPG #3:35, "Depression (Psychiatric)."
- <u>Prognosis</u> of an individual manic-depressive episode is good, even without treatment, provided that the patient does not suffer from complete physical exhaustion in the manic phase, or commit suicide in the depressive phase. Manic-depressive illness is a self-limiting condition which may

recur, as opposed to the chronic deterioration of schizophrenia.
- <u>Treatment aims</u> are to eliminate the extremes of the mood swings; lithium carbonate is frequently used for this purpose. Tranquilizers are given to control hyperactivity and ECT may be used. Once the immediate psychotic state has improved, psychotherapy is utilized to enhance functioning and level of wellness. See NCPG's #3:46, "Drugs: Psychotropic," and 3:47, "Drugs: Tranquilizers."
- <u>Nursing Responsibilities</u> include: manipulating the environment to meet the patient's needs, working with patient to identify and resolve painful feelings, teaching patient regarding medications and planning for discharge.

Specific Considerations, Potential Patient Outcomes and Nursing Actions:

1) Hyperactivity, Verbal and Motor

The patient will demonstrate increased ability to control motor and verbal behaviors:
- assess motor & verbal behaviors as unobtrusively as possible, and set limits PRN;
- know that important cues for setting limits are: a care giver is worried about potential suicide; feels that pt. is saying, "please take over. . .;" or patient is upsetting self and/or others with own behavior;
- remove pt. from all stimulating, exciting, noisy, disturbing influences, while still providing ample space for him to move around; explain firmly and quietly that a staff member will stay with him while he paces, talks, etc.; engage in conversation with pt. as little as possible; let him know that the therapeutic plan is to de-escalate the hyperactivity and to provide a quiet, safe place for him.
- assess if pt. is a danger to himself or others: ask him specifically if he has any suicidal or homicidal thoughts; if "yes," report to Dr., and ensure that pt. is staffed on a 1-to-1 basis (see NCPG #3:38, "The Suicidal Patient;")
- be alert to pt's. wish to leave hospital (most manic patients do not see the need for hospitalization, or the danger to themselves); if pt. not on 1-to-1, have him stay within sight of staff;
- promote rest & sleep by limiting exciting influences, giving warm bath, back rub, etc.; give sedatives as ordered.

2) Loss of Interest in Self-Care

Patient will carry out own personal hygiene and grooming:
- see nursing actions for consideration #6 ("Loss of Interest in Self-Care") in NCPG #3:37, "Schizophrenia."

3) "Flight of Ideas" (Related to Associative Looseness)

The patient will be able to communicate clearly with staff:
- see nursing actions for consideration #3 ("Associative Looseness") in NCPG #3:37, "Schizophrenia."

4) Unrealistic, Grandiose Ideas

The patient will express realtistic ideas and plans:
- do not talk to pt. about the grandiose ideas, as that is non-therapeutic and pt. may become more out of control; rather, provide limits with a quiet room, walking or talking quietly, keeping in mind that the pt. is experiencing feelings of being overwhelmed;

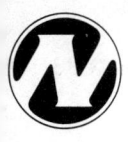

The Patient with Manic-Depressive Psychosis

    - look for the reality stimuli causing the stress, and explore this with pt.; interpret reality for him by telling him you feel he must be very anxious right now... and listen for any feeling tone in his response, following up on it.

5) Inability to Cope with Painful Feelings (Grief, Guilt, Sadness, Anger)
The patient will identify and talk about the painful feelings he is experiencing:
- know that patient's inability to cope with painful feelings comes to the foreground as manic behavior begins to lessen;
- see nursing actions for consideration #1 ("Inability to Cope with Painful Feelings") in NCPG #3:35, "Depression."

6) Depressive Behaviors   Read NCPG #3:35, "Depression 'Psychiatric'") and NCPG #3:38, "The Suicidal Patient."

Discharge Planning and Teaching Objectives/Outcomes:
1) (Patient and/or family/significant other) Can identify feelings, behaviors indicative of an approaching manic-depressive episode and knows to contact Dr., or clinic when this occurs.
2) Knows importance of expressing feelings to others in order to facilitate communication & understanding & to receive support during difficult times.
3) Can perform personal hygiene and grooming activities on a daily basis.
4) Can take own medicines, knows the purpose and potential side effects of each and to call doctor/clinic if these occur. Has a supply of medicines, and knows how to obtain refills.

Recommended References
- "Drugs: Hypnotics & Sedatives," NCP Guide #3:45.
- "Drugs: Psychotropic," NCP Guide #3:46.
- "Drugs: Tranquilizers," NCP Guide #3:47.
- "Mood Swings," by B. Befner, *Nursing '72*, August, 1972: 28-31.
- "The Patient Experiencing Depression (Psychiatric)," NCP Guide #3:35.
- "The Patient with Schizophrenia," NCP Guide #3:37.
- "The Patient who is Suicidal (on a Psychiatric Unit)," NCP Guide #3:38.

©Margo Creighton Neal, 1977

NCP Guide No. **3:36** 66

The Patient Manifesting Manipulation

Definition: The process of influencing another in such a way that one meets his own needs and wishes without regard to the needs, wishes, and functions of others.

LONG TERM GOAL: The patient will be able to express his needs and wishes in such a way that he demonstrates responsibility for his own actions and does not cause harm to others.

General Considerations:
— **Manipulation is a method** utilized by all persons to attempt to have the world come out as they want it. When manipulation is no longer seen as being acceptable because of the method or level, then it is perceived by others as negative and antisocial.
— Lifelong patterns of behavior are difficult to change and change only occurs if something else replaces the behavior; this new behavior must be perceived as rewarded and pleasurable.
— **Nursing assessment** includes a knowledge of the behavioral manifestations of manipulation which include: (1) pretends to be helpless; (2) pits staff, nurses, doctors against each other; (3) insincere complimenting of a staff member to her face, followed by negative comments about her to others; (4) makes undefined, ongoing demands; (5) makes excessive, unnecessary demands for staff time; (6) presents self as lonely and distraught in order to keep staff with him; this behavior continues to occur with no apparent resolution, even when intervention has occurred; (7) continues to act out (demand, yell, complain, etc.) even when repeatedly told that this is unacceptable behavior. Assessment also includes an awareness of the function and rewards of this behavior for the patient.
— **Nursing responsibilities** include reinforcing reality and preventing manipulation of self and others by the patient. Written, clear nursing care plans are the best tools to do this. Interventions should be based on principles of reinforcement theory.

Specific Considerations, Potential Patient Outcomes, and Nursing Actions:

1) Immediate Response to Recognition of Manipulation

The patient will verbally acknowledge that his present behavior is socially unacceptable and possibly physically harmful to himself and/or others:
— confront the pt. with his attempts at manipulation, then ignore manipulative behavior when possible;
— give praise, positive feedback & rewards such as social interaction, visitors, for non-manipulative behavior;
— allow the verbal expression of angry feelings;
— set limits on destructive behavior;
— tell the pt. to deal directly with you, otherwise you will continue to confront him with the efforts of manipulation;
— accurately record the instruction & information you give the pt. in the nursing notes & nursing care plans; this approach is useful in discouraging the pt. from changing, ignoring or distorting the communication;

— keep family informed of what you are doing & why.

2) Restoration to Adaptive Coping

The patient will accept responsibility for his actions, will be actively involved in his care and will accept the positive responses of others:
- plan nursing care plans & daily routine with pt.;
- decide who (pt. or nurse) is responsible for exactly what care, communicate this arrangement to staff, both verbally and in written plan;
- evaluate results of nursing care with the pt.;
- praise the pt.'s efforts in carrying out his responsibilities;
- accompany the Dr. on rounds to discourage the pt.'s distortion & misuse of what the Dr. has told him;
- clear, consistent communication among staff at all levels about the pt.'s manipulative behavior & the approach to be utilized is extremely important;
- praise staff & family members for their efforts at reducing the manipulative behavior of the pt.

Discharge Planning and Teaching Objectives/Outcomes
1) (Patient/Family/Significant Other) Can verbalize the way in which undesired manipulative behavior was being expressed.
2) Can accept the positive feedback for socially acceptable behavior.
3) Can ask directly for the needs to be met, questions answered.
4) Can wait for answers, needs to be met when the situation/need is not an emergency.

Recommended References
"Alienation" by Dorothy Block in Carlson, Carolyn and Blackwell, Betty, *Behavioral Concepts and Nursing Interventions*. Philadelphia: J.B. Lippincott Co., 1978:116–127.
"A Systematic Approach to the Evaluation of Interpersonal Relationships," by Linda Aiken and James Aiken. *American Journal of Nursing*, May 1973:863.
"Coping With a Seductive Patient." *Nursing '78*, July 1978:40–45.
"Debbie Got Attention the Hard Way," by Diana Guthrie. *Nursing '75*, November 1975:52–54.
"Mrs. Myers Played the Buzzer Game," by Joyce Kee. *Nursing '76*, July 1976:14–16.
"Two Types of Problem Patients . . . and How to Deal With Them," by Gertrude Ujhely. *Nursing '76*, July 1976:64–67.
"When It Comes to Difficult Patients, Mr. Billman Was a Showstopper," by Patricia Sharer. *Nursing '77*, September 1977:36–37.

© Margo Creighton Neal, 1980

The Patient Manifesting Noncompliance

Definition: Noncompliance in a health care setting means not adhering (or only partially adhering) to a prescribed therapeutic or disease-prevention regimen.

LONG TERM GOAL: The patient will comply with prescribed treatment or prevention regimen in a responsible, informed manner; the patient will be assisted to participate adequately in self-care and achieve maximum health potential.

General Considerations:
- **Behavioral manifestations** of noncompliance include:
  - disregards suggested health regimen
  - cooperates with some parts but does not adhere to rest of care plan
  - "forgets" appointments, medications, treatments
  - affect is distrustful, angry, fearful
  - anxiety
  - continuously postpones health care
- **Causes** can include:
  - lack of understanding of diagnosis and treatment plan
  - denial of illness and consequences
  - life-style of continual crisis
  - desire to remain ill and dependent for secondary gains
  - low self-esteem
  - home or job demands
  - cost of treatment
  - negative attitude toward health care providers
  - high stress level
  - severe symptoms due to prescribed treatment
- Compliance is enhanced by use of teaching programs, by a positive and accepting attitude on the part of health professionals, and by efforts to stimulate patient and family motivation.
- **Nursing responsibilities include** assessment of variables affecting patient's compliance and noncompliance behaviors in order to recognize and support positive coping mechanisms and achieve participation and cooperation in health care.

Specific Considerations, Potential Patient Outcomes, and Nursing Actions:

1) Immediate Response to Recognition of Noncompliance

The patient will be able to discuss situation in which s/he was noncompliant; the patient will be accepted and valued as a unique individual:
— listen attentively to pt.'s ideas & concerns; allow pt. to describe situation from his point of view; assess reality perception;
— treat pt. in respectful way; approach in unhurried, relaxed manner; avoid negative criticism;

- encourage expression of feelings, i.e., "Tell me more about your concerns with the side effects of your blood pressure medication;"
- summarize & reflect back expressions of feelings, i.e., "So you're saying you were really upset/scared/angry when you heard the results of your blood test;"
- encourage pt. to define & discuss own needs; refrain from forcing treatments;
- assess for stress level, stage of loss, anxiety, negative attitudes towards health professionals, self-esteem (see recommended references);
- see NCPGs #1:21, "The Patient Manifesting Anger," #1:22, "The Patient Manifesting Anxiety," #1:24, "The Patient Manifesting Denial," & #1:28, "The Patient Experiencing Fear."

2) Restoration to Adaptive Coping

The patient will accept information about prescribed therapeutic plan; the patient will be an active participant in planning and implementing care plan; the patient will participate in self-care:
- ask questions to assess pt.'s knowledge of diagnosis, disease process, treatment plan, & specific treatments;
- explore with pt. the effects of his behavior of noncompliance on self & significant others (SOs);
- encourage mutual problem solving & interdependence; explain team approach with pt. as an important part of team;
- assess problem-solving skills & teach as needed; see NCPG #5:47, "Problem Solving;"
- invite pt. to ask questions; provide reliable information; see NCPG #1:49, "Teaching Patients: General Suggestions;"
- discuss & explain procedures in advance; do not surprise pt., prepare pt. for new situations by anticipating situation & utilizing role playing, problem solving, & behavior modification;
- give verbal & non-verbal positive reinforcement for adaptive coping & appropriate compliance;
- involve pt. in active participation in setting goals & planning care; involve family & SOs as pt. desires;
- invite pt. to express preferences, likes & dislikes as much as possible in the situation;
- encourage pt. to participate in activities of daily living (ADL) in his own way; praise for participation in self-care;
- be aware that cost of medication or treatment is often a problem for elderly, adolescents, & heads of household; make appropriate referral to social service as needed;
- consult with physician & other health team members to explore problems & plan pt. care;
- refrain from performing nonessential procedures;
- introduce pt. to other persons who have had similar experiences & have positive reactions.

Discharge Planning and Teaching Objectives/Outcomes
1) (Patient/Family/Significant Other) Can approach health professionals for consultation in health maintenance and health care.
2) Can ask for information about treatment plan, can express feelings and concerns about treatment plan.
3) Is able to explain reason for and intended effect of treatments.
4) States s/he will cooperate with treatment plan in a responsible, informed, active way.
5) Can describe dangerous effects of poor health practices, of noncompliance with prescribed regimen.

Recommended References
"Behavior Modification." *NCP Guide #5:37,* Nurseco, 1981.
"The Patient Experiencing Anger." *NCP Guide #1:21,* 2nd Ed., Nurseco, 1980.
"The Patient Experiencing Anxiety." *NCP Guide #1:22,* 2nd Ed., Nurseco, 1980.
"The Patient Experiencing Denial." *NCP Guide #1:24,* 2nd Ed., Nurseco, 1980.
"The Patient Experiencing A Threat to Self-Esteem." *NCP Guide #5:32,* Nurseco, 1981.
"Problem Solving." *NCP Guide #5:47,* Nurseco, 1981.
"Responses to Loss: The Grief and Mourning Process." *NCP Guide #1:31,* 2nd Ed., Nurseco, 1980.
"Stress Management." *NCP Guide #5:49,* Nurseco, 1981.
"Teaching Patients: General Suggestions." *NCP Guide #1:49,* 2nd Ed., Nurseco, 1980.

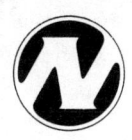

The Patient Experiencing Pain

Definition: Pain is a situation that is the result of a single or class of stimuli; when perceived, it is accompanied by emotional and/or physical reactions.

LONG TERM GOAL: The patient will be free of pain and/or discomfort which impairs day to day functioning and the accomplishment of life goals.

General Considerations:
— **Pain** is the result of perception of noxious stimuli. The perception of pain is a protective mechanism and involves the nerve endings, spinal cord, brain stem, and cerebral cortex. The stimuli can be (1) *mechanical* (blow, friction), (2) *chemical* (microorganism, toxins, drugs), (3) *thermal* (hot and cold) or (4) *electrical current*.
— **Pain** can be (1) *superficial:* involves the cutaneous receptors, is localized, and has a sharp quality; (2) *deep:* from muscles, viscera; is more persistent, usually dull in nature and more diffuse; (3) *referred:* usually occurs at visceral level but actual point of focus of reaction or perception of pain is away from area of occurrence, eg. pain in an ischemic heart is felt in lower chest and/or left arm.
— **Pain threshold is based on several variables,** including: (1) type of pain stimuli, (2) location of pain stimuli, (3) cultural practices, (4) previous experience with pain in same or other body locations, (5) general body health and patient's perception of own health, (6) emotional health and fears associated with pain, and (7) source of pain: internal (body defense reaction) or external (clothing, dressings, position, noise).
— **Nursing assessment** includes observing for behavioral and physiological manifestations of pain which include: (1) pulse and blood pressure changes, (2) respiratory changes, (3) excessive perspiration, (4) nausea and vomiting, (5) changes in skin color, (6) generalized or localized muscle tension, (7) restlessness and tremor, (8) clenched fists, (9) spasm and muscle aches, (10) mood changes, (11) restlessness, (12) fear, (13) anxiety, (14) aggression, (15) impatience, (16) change in facial expression, (17) crying, groaning, grunting or gasping.
— **Nursing responsibilities** include knowledge of up-to-date treatment and prevention of pain, and an awareness of the fact that each individual has a different response to pain. *Intervention* should be directed toward relief of acute pain or treatment and reduction of chronic pain.

Specific Considerations, Potential Patient Outcomes, and Nursing Actions:

1) Immediate Response to Recognition of Pain

The patient will verbalize the feeling of reduction or alleviation of pain:
— determine the pt.'s pain history, previous responses as well as present ones;
— encourage the pt. to talk about his experiences with pain by showing interest in what he is saying, e.g. make eye contact, nod your head at times to respond to him, & especially, sit down with him when he is sharing feelings with you;
— utilize the knowledge you have about the pt.'s reaction & tolerance to pain as well as the doctor's orders to make your decisions about giving medication; do not withhold medication just because you feel the pt.'s pain is not real or should be adequately tolerated; remember . . . it is the pt. who is feeling the pain; there is suffering going on whether or not the pain exists or varies in level;
— when giving pain medication, tell the pt. about the medication & its expected effect; talk positively about it;
— utilize activities & conversation to help the pt. focus on something other than the pain; find out what s/he likes to talk about and/or activities s/he enjoys;
— do not reinforce the focus on pain in someone with chronic pain; instead, use behavior modification techniques & begin to reward non-pain focused behavior.

2) Restoration to Adaptive Coping

The patient will be able to distinguish between pain-related and non-pain-related activities; will engage in activities without constant thought of pain and will respond to reinforcement of non-pain-related living by making future life plans:
— plan with the pt. the kinds & timing of activities that can reduce, eliminate or minimize the suffering;
— pts. in pain cannot tolerate being rushed; when pt. is caring for self, allow as much time as s/he need to accomplish the task;
— allow the pt. to talk intermittently about the pain & suffering but not constantly; finding the cause of the suffering often relieves or reduces it;
— give positive feedback to the pt.'s efforts to share feelings & cope with the suffering;
— have friends, family, & staff available to pt. when s/he needs them;
— make sure all staff is aware of the pt.'s usual response to pain;
— hold pt. care conferences to discuss pt.'s responses to pain; plan approaches & write them in nursing care plan;
— take a few seconds & inwardly ask yourself, "What would I be like if I were suffering like this pt.?" Remember . . . identification of how we feel & respond increases our understanding of the variety of ways other people respond to situations, particularly painful experiences;
— facilitate significant others' understanding of the pt.'s suffering by giving careful explanations to them of how & why the pt. responds as s/he does;
— attempt to understand the religious, cultural & psychological influences in patterns of this particular pt.'s reaction to pain;

- teach pt. body relaxation techniques that can be utilized not only for pain reduction but during periods of tension & anxiety (these periods can elicit tension & anxiety in pain perception & reaction);
- teach pt. to use medication, support systems, diversional therapy & relaxation to cope with pain;
- for chronic pain, the patient should not only be aware of use of relaxation, behavioral & diversional therapy, but should have knowledge of outside resources such as pain clinics, reputable hypnotists & acupuncturists; refer PRN.

Discharge Planning and Teaching Objectives/Outcomes
1) (Patient/Family/Significant Other) Can verbalize events and conditions which influence the occurrence and level of pain.
2) Can identify medication use, diversional and relaxation activities that assist in the reduction or elimination of pain.
3) Can name community resources available for the ongoing treatment of intractable pain.
4) Can verbalize emotional responses to constant focusing on pain.

Recommended References
"Analgesics at the Bedside," by Nessa Coyle. *American Journal of Nursing*, September 1979:1554–1557.
"Angina: Teach Your Patients to Prevent Recurrent Attacks," by C. Walton and B. Hammond. *Nursing '78*, February 1978:32–38.
"Assessing Pain," by Ada Jacox. *American Journal of Nursing*, May 1979:895–900.
"Helping Patients Overcome the Disabling Effects of Chronic Pain," by J. Blair Pace. *Nursing '77*, July 1977:38–43.
"McGill-Melzack Pain Questionnaire," by Judith E. Meissner. *Nursing '80*, January 1980:50-51.
Nursing Management of the Patient with Pain, by M. McCaffery. Philadelphia: J.B. Lippincott Co., 1972.
"Pain and Suffering—A Special Supplement." *American Journal of Nursing*, March 1974:489.
"The Management of Pain: Using Analgesics Effectively," by M. DiBlasi and C. Washburn. *American Journal of Nursing*, January 1979:74–78.
"The Patient in Pain: New Concepts," by Jeanne Benoliel and Dorothy Crowley. *Nursing Digest*, Summer 1977:41–48.

© Margo Creighton Neal, 1980

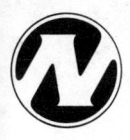

The Patient Experiencing Powerlessness

Definition: Powerlessness is a perceived lack of personal power or control over life events and experiences in a specific situation.

LONG TERM GOAL: The patient will experience an increased sense of power and control over life events and experiences.

General Considerations:
- **Personal power** comes from being capable, adequate and able to master the environment.
- **Powerlessness results from loss of control** over environment, self-functioning, or own behavior, and **lack of knowledge** regarding own illness or life experience, including the implications for here-and-now and future for self, family, or significant other. Loss of control may involve psychological and physiological variables.
- **Potential causes** of powerlessness include:
  - diagnosis of acute or chronic illness with disability and loss of control over body, mental ability, and independent role;
  - being a "patient" instead of usual "well" person;
  - hospitalization;
  - emergency admission due to accident or sudden acute symptoms;
  - admission to CCU or ICU;
  - developmental change with potential loss of function and abilities as in aging, or change in function and abilities as in adolescence and menopause;
  - interpersonal and relationship problems, e.g. divorce, separation, termination of a relationship, family problems;
  - actual or potential loss of significant other by death, illness, divorce, or separation; potential loss of own life due to disease process or accident;
  - dealing with insurance companies, social security, and other large organizations upon which one may be dependent for help;
  - low self-esteem, situational or chronic;
  - perception of authority figure as distant, unapproachable, talking in technical terms, non-available, not interested, not responsive.

- **Behavioral manifestations** of powerlessness include:
  - frustration, discouragement
  - anger, hostility
  - withdrawal
  - passivity
  - depression
  - loss of perspective
  - fear
  - sadness, crying
  - denial
  - asks many questions
  - asks no questions
  - inability to carry out activities of daily living
  - confusion
  - inability to learn
  - inability to concentrate
  - defensive coping mechanisms
- **Nursing responsibilities** include an awareness of potential causes, recognition of behaviors, and prescribing interventions to assist the patient to adapt to current life situation in a way that will enhance his sense of power and control.

Specific Considerations, Potential Patient Outcomes, and Nursing Actions:

1) Immediate Response to Recognition of Powerlessness

    The patient will express feelings and concerns about situations in which s/he feels powerless:
    — build a trust relationship by making frequent verbal & nonverbal contact with pt.; be consistent & dependable (see NCPGs #1:21, "Patient Manifesting Anger," #1:22, "Patient Experiencing Confusion," #1:24, "Patient Manifesting Denial," #1:28, "Patient Experiencing Fear");
    — listen to pt.'s feelings & concerns;
    — ask the pt. for his opinions, likes, dislikes, & wishes; utilize these in making care plan;
    — ensure environmental *powerfulness* by putting call light, telephone, bedside stand, urinal, & other desired items within reach; be aware that hospital room & objects in it are pt.'s territory & respect his right to exert control over it.

2) Restoration of Control and Power

    The patient will identify situation in which s/he feels powerless; the patient will problem solve, set goals, and try alternative adaptive behaviors to increase sense of control and power:
    — promote active participation in simple & appropriate decision making in ADL such as diet preferences, time & type of hygiene measures, arrangement of physical surroundings;
    — assist pt. to identify situations in which s/he feels powerless; let pt. describe situation as s/he sees it;
    — provide situations in which the pt. can take control (e.g., "Would you prefer to have your dressing changed before or after lunch?" or "Would you like us to block the telephone until you're ready to receive calls?" or "How would you like your bedside stand arranged?");
    — give pt. verbal & non-verbal positive reinforcement & acknowledgment for active participation in planning care in ADL, goal

setting, & alternative behaviors which increase sense of power & control (e.g. verbally acknowledge that pt. made a list of questions to ask physician, asked the questions, & clarified information; or, "I see you can do your own colostomy care; how do you feel about that?" or "You have some good ideas on how to manage at home; would you like to discuss them with the discharge planning nurse?"); see NCPG #5:37, "Behavior Modification;"
— assess for readiness to assume more complicated decision making; influencing factors include severity & stability of disease process (pt. in crisis or with acute symptoms may only be able to participate in a few simple decisions), previous coping mechanisms, ability to problem solve, personality traits (passive or non-assertive persons may not know how to problem solve or make decisions); these data should be assessed before offering pt. more complicated choices; when pt. ready, utilize chart & family members to facilitate situations in which pt. can achieve increased power & control;
— assess pt.'s perception & knowledge of treatments, treatment program, diagnosis & symptoms; encourage him to express his views *before* giving information, explanation, or reassurance (e.g., "What has your doctor told you about your new medication? How do you feel about taking it? What do you expect to happen in x-ray tomorrow? How do you see yourself getting up to the bathroom at home? What do you think works the best for your back pain?");
— know that increased knowledge leads to increased sense of power; assess for learning needs & provide information PRN; see NCPGs #1:49, 50, "Teaching Patients;"
— assess pt.'s ability to problem solve & health teach as needed; include significant other & family as pt. desires; see NCPG #5:47, "Problem Solving;"
— assist pt. to direct & plan own care within the medical treatment plan; as much as safely possible, allow pt. to decide how the nurse & other health team members will participate;
— encourage pt. to ask questions; be able to say, "I don't know, but I'm willing to find out" or "I don't know; this is where you can find out;"
— assess communication patterns; assist pt. to identify own preferences, likes & dislikes, wants, feelings, values, & attitudes; reinforce clear, assertive communication of preferences & feelings to appropriate listeners; let pt. know that s/he has a choice of content & person with whom s/he communicates.

Discharge Planning and Teaching Objectives/Outcomes
1) (Patient/Family/Significant Other) Verbalizes situations in which s/he feels powerless.
2) Can describe own behaviors which enhance sense of power and control.
3) States s/he will use situational supports to take an active role in own health care.

Recommended References

"ANA Code for Nurses Revised for Greater Focus on Nurse and Client," by R.D. Hadley. *American Nurse*, October 15, 1976.
"Behavior Modification." *NCP Guide #5:37,* Nurseco, 1981.
Patient Problems in Self-Esteem and Nursing Interventions, by Merle Mishel. Los Angeles: California State University Press, 1976:61–64.
"The Patient Experiencing Confusion." *NCP Guide #1:23,* 2nd Ed., Nurseco, 1980.
"The Patient Experiencing Fear." *NCP Guide #1:28,* 2nd Ed., Nurseco, 1980.
"The Patient Manifesting Anger." *NCP Guide #1:21,* 2nd Ed., Nurseco, 1980.
"The Patient Manifesting Denial." *NCP Guide #1:24,* 2nd Ed., Nurseco, 1980.
"Problem Solving." *NCP Guide #5:47,* Nurseco, 1981.
"Teaching Patients: General Suggestions." *NCP Guide #1:49,* 2nd Ed., Nurseco, 1980.
"Teaching Patients: Specific Plan for Skills and Procedures." *NCP Guide #1:50,* 2nd Ed., Nurseco, 1980.

NCP Guide No. **4:39** **81**

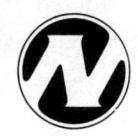

The Adult Victim of <u>Rape/Sexual Assault</u> (in the ER)

Definition: Rape is any forced sexual activity. The legal definition refers to forced, vaginal penetration. Other forced sexual acts may be referred to as sexual assaults.

LONG TERM GOAL: The victim will regain her emotional, physical, social and sexual equilibrium.

General Considerations:
- <u>Incidence</u>: a woman is raped approximately Q 2 mins. in the U.S.; only about 10% of all rapes are reported. Although men, women and children are raped, most rapes and sexual assaults are committed by men against women.
- The <u>result</u> of rape for the victim is the disruption of her physical, emotional, social and sexual equilibrium. The rape is a situational hazard and a true emotional crisis may or may not occur, depending upon the victim's coping mechanisms and available sources of support. (The way a victim is treated in ER by police, courts, family, can often be the "last straw" that pushes her into an actual crisis.) Refer to NCPG #2:31, "Crisis Intervention."
- The <u>psychological impact</u> is severe, may be long lasting & is significantly affected by the type of immediate care the victim receives.
- In the past, <u>research & attention</u> have focused primarily on the rapist; now, due largely to efforts and research by women, the focus is on the victim and her ensuing disequilibrium.
- Many <u>myths</u> are perpetrated about rape but the <u>realities</u> are far different:
    - <u>myth</u>: Women "lead men on" and "ask for it" by their dress & behavior.
    - <u>reality</u>: Most rapes are planned by the rapist and are not provoked by dress or behavior. Ask yourself how young children or 80+ year-old women might have dressed or behaved.
    - <u>myth</u>: Most rapes are spontaneous & unplanned.
    - <u>reality</u>: Most rapists have observed their victim's living patterns and planned the attack.
    - <u>myth</u>: Rapists are usually strangers to their victims.
    - <u>reality</u>: Most rapists are in some way acquainted with their victims, either casually or fairly well-known.
    - <u>myth</u>: Most rapes are racial and are usually done by black men against white women.
    - <u>reality</u>: Most rapes are <u>intra-racial</u>; one study showed that 70% of all urban rapes were committed by black men on black women.
    - <u>myth</u>: Rape is a sex crime.
    - <u>reality</u>: No, it is a crime of violence and power in which the rapist gets emotional, and usually sexual, gratification from physical dominance

and control over a powerless victim.
- *myth*: Rape is a non-violent crime.
- *reality*: It is a violent crime, usually carried out under threat of death.
- *myth*: Many women will consent to sexual intercourse then cry "rape" out of revenge or hysteria.
- *reality*: Only about 2% of all rape and related sex charges are found to be false—about the same percent as other felonies.
- *myth*: Women secretly want to be raped.
- *reality*: Some women do fantasize about rape, but usually as aggressive sex, and not for what it really is: a terrifying, brutalizing & humiliating experience. Rape is not sex by consensus.
- *myth*: It could never happen to me.
- *reality*: All women are potential rape victims, regardless of age, race, circumstances, dress, physical attributes.
- *myth*: Rape is motivated by sexual needs.
- *reality*: Most rapists have other sexual partners, have normal personalities and are much like most men you meet, only with a greater tendency to express violence and rage.

- **The Emergency room (ER) experience** can be either a calming, supportive one or one in which the victim experiences further injustice from the ER staff due to professional insensitivity & unhelpful attitudes:
    - ER staff often question, "Was she _really_ raped?" and put blame and responsibility on the victim. Frequently, this is because the staff person is made aware of own vulnerability to rape when confronted with a victim, and the situation is understandably anxiety-producing.
    - Research shows that typical reactions of rape victims in ER are either "expressed" such as crying, laughing, nervousness; or "controlled", e.g. outward calm. If a victim is exhibiting the latter behavior, there is a tendency among ER staff to feel she has not been raped, or is dealing with it so well that she needs no help.
    - Staff often experience feelings of being overwhelmed by victim and not knowing what to do.
    - ER staff should realize that the victim has just emerged from a terrifying experience and is _not responsible_ for what was done to her; the rapist is responsible for the attack. When ER staff can understand this and act accordingly, they have an excellent opportunity to help alleviate the trauma inherent in the ER experience itself, and help the victim regain her equilibrium and potentially prevent future psychological problems.
- **Goals of medical treatment** are: to prevent infection, VD & pregnancy, and to collect physical evidence.
- **The ER nurse's responsibilities are**: to _believe_ what victim says; to _provide_ basic crisis intervention techniques; to _provide_ for immediate safety needs of victim; to _provide & assist_ with medical treatment needs; to _collect & prepare evidence_ for the police; to _provide_ community referral resources; to _be aware of own feelings & attitudes_ and their effect on contact with victim; and _to do anticipatory guidance_ with victim and family/SO.

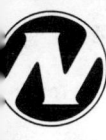

The Adult Victim of Rape/Sexual Assault (in the ER)

Specific Considerations, Potential Patient Outcomes and Nursing Actions:

Acute Physical & Emotional Reaction to Rape Trauma

The victim will receive situational support from staff and be allowed to cope with situation in her own way; will regain a measure of control over her life space; will receive appropriate medical treatment:

- always provide a private examining room;
- listen to what the victim is saying (this will help her regain control) & believe what she says (ER is not the place to be judgmental); acknowledge the assault, encourage her to talk & be supportive of her, e.g. "It must have been a terrifying ordeal for you...;" express warmth, interest, respect & a non-judgmental attitude; allow open ventilation of feelings, especially anger at the rapist; be aware that this anger may be directed at staff;
- ask her what is the most difficult thing for her right now & discuss it with her, refraining from giving advice or "You should have...," or "Why did you...?" (such statements will not be helpful); provide whatever victim wants & needs to help lower her stress, e.g. information, privacy, kleenex, warm covers, coffee, etc.;
- if she says "It was my fault," or "I should have..."—reinforce that the attack was not her fault, but the fault of the rapist & that she did what she was forced to do in order to save her life; (many victims "pay" the rapist for their life with the sexual act, then feel guilty, unclean, ashamed, self-critical);
- encourage victim to talk about her feelings of the experience, usually of overwhelming terror, but do not dwell on the sexual aspects;
- victim may not wish to talk and/or may look undisturbed, or seem to be coping extremely well; may be denying or minimizing the attack; if any of these, allow her to cope in this way but tell her that at a later date, she may experience feelings of anger, fear or sadness, and that this would be a usual reaction;
- do all interviewing sensitively & with consideration for victim's feelings; while it will be necessary (for court records) to know the explicit sexual acts involved, only one person needs to do this once (either Dr. or nurse) others can read it in the chart;
- have a female staff member be with victim at all times, to be her advocate, especially during any examination or interrogation; if your hospital has a rape team, a member may fulfill this function; if victim asks for a female police officer, make all attempts to comply with request;
- assess victim's ability to cope: what is her level of anxiety? her perception of what occurred? does she have available family/significant other (SO) outside the hospital? what is her emotional response?

- express your belief in her ability to deal with problems/decisions she will face in next few days; be sure she takes an active role in making & carrying out plans, e.g. reporting to police, returning to work, etc.
- assist with collection of physical evidence; read NCPG #4:46;
- if victim is alone, & she consents, call her family/SO & ask them to bring a change of clothes for her; if she has no one to call, develop a safety plan for her, e.g. transportation home;
- provide her with information about available counseling services, options, rights & follow-up treatments; allow her to use telephone to call crisis/rape center.

2) Reaction of Family/SOs to the Victim's Experience

Family/SOs will verbalize an understanding of what victim has experienced; will give client situational support:
- assess family/SO's reaction to the victim's situation; be aware that they often tend to blame the victim, to be non-supportive & to isolate her; reinforce to them that the attack was <u>not the victim's fault</u> or responsibility & that it was a <u>terrifying</u> experience in which she was afraid she would be killed, that whatever her response to the rapist was, it was a decision made to try to save her life or prevent bodily harm to herself and/or to her children;
- family/SOs may feel they are responsible because they weren't there to protect victim and thus feel guilty & vulnerable; again, emphasize that the responsibility <u>lies with the attacker</u>;
- assess & discuss with them ways they can be supportive to victim, e.g. by listening to & believing what victim says; encouraging & allowing victim to talk; helping victim to resume her usual life activities; not over-protecting her; letting victim make the decision to prosecute or not; not dwelling on the sexual part of the rape, but on the victim's <u>feelings</u>, usually ones of overwhelming terror; stress that victim needs to be held & stroked just as she would in any stressful situation & not to withhold touch (otherwise, they may reinforce victim's feelings of being unclean, ruined);
- share with them that it is typical that rape victims will have increasing fear & anxiety during next 48 hours, and may want to talk at length about the experience; that victim may then "seem" to adjust, but may re-experience the feelings of the attack at a later date;
- tell them that victim may not want to talk about the assault, & if so, they should not press her but continue to provide caring & support;
- tell them to work out with victim ways for her to <u>be</u> & <u>feel</u> safe, e.g. locks on windows, new lights, not walking alone at night, etc. some action may need to be taken immediately, e.g. changing locks;
- assess SO's coping; often they are the ones to go into crisis & need a mental health referral for themselves; assess victim's equilibrium after she sees family/SO.

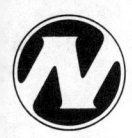

The Adult Victim of Rape/Sexual Assault (in the ER)

Discharge Planning and Teaching Objectives/Outcomes:
1) Victim has someone to leave ER with, does not have to go home alone.
2) Has a referral and/or contact with a mental health counselor. Has resources or referral to a Dr./clinic for follow-up physical care.
3) Knows how to use prescribed medications, and symptoms/reactions to watch for.

Recommended References
"An Interagency Service Network to Meet Needs of Rape Victims," by Grace Hardgrove, Social Casework, April 1976: 245-253.
"Care of the Rape Victim in Emergency," by Sandra LeFort, The Canadian Nurse, February 1977: 42-45.
"Coping Behavior of the Rape Victim," by Ann W. Burgess & Lynda L. Holmstrom, American Journal of Psychiatry, April 1976: 413-417.
"Crisis and Counseling Requests of Rape Victims," by Ann W. Burgess & Lynda L. Holmstrom, Nursing Research, May-June 1974: 196-202.
"Evidence Collection: Rape/Sexual Assault," NCP Guide #4:46, Nurseco, 1978.
"Learn to Fight Rape Without Hang-ups," by Irene Horoshak, RN, July 1976: 52-56.
"The Patient Needing Crisis Intervention," NCP Guide #2:31, Nurseco, 1975.
"Rape: a Plea for Help in the Hospital Emergency Room," by Cindy C. Williams & Reg A. Williams, Nursing Forum Fall 1973: 388-401.

© Margo Creighton Neal, 1978

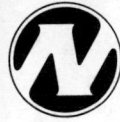

The Patient with <u>Schizophrenia</u>

Definition: Schizophrenia is a psychotic reaction, manifested by fundamental disturbances in a person's interactions with people, and ability to think and and communicate clearly.

LONG TERM GOAL: The patient will regain some measure of independence in self-care, take own medicines, and demonstrate increased ability to communicate with others.

General Considerations:
- <u>Incidence</u>: Schizophrenia is a complex psychiatric problem, accounting for approximately one-half of the population in mental hospitals. Most persons with symptomatology of schizophrenia are able to maintain themselves in society and are never hospitalized.
- <u>Onset</u> occurs most frequently between the ages of 17 and 27. There are several theories of etiology and research in this area is continuing.
- <u>Acute vs. chronic</u>: The course of schizophrenia varies: some patients have an acute break with reality, respond quickly to treatment and are able to resume their life. Some begin to withdraw slowly and become steadily less in touch with reality. Others begin with an acute stage, decrease symptoms while in the hospital and then resume symptoms whenever stress increases. The latter course tends to become a chronic symptom pattern.
- <u>Types</u>: (1) <u>paranoid</u> - manifested by extreme suspiciousness and delusions; may feel that people are against him or that voices are threatening him or telling him to do dangerous or violent acts. Also may state that he believes he is Christ or some important figure.
  (2) <u>catatonic</u> - manifested by abnormal postural movements: in extreme cases, patient may become so inactive that he cannot move, take care of himself or talk; this is called "catatonic stupor." At the other extreme, he may go into "catatonic excitement," manifested by excessive motor activity and extreme agitation; the patient does not eat or sleep and may become dehydrated and exhausted.
  (3) <u>simple</u> - manifested by total lack of any substantial relationships, lack of social skills, apathy; no overt delusions, hallucinations or illusions.
  (4) <u>hebrephrenic</u> - manifested by inappropriate affect, giggling, unrelated smiling and laughter and regression to an earlier period of life. May have grandiose delusions and hallucinations. Often has disregard of social restrictions; may dress bizarrely, urinate and defecate at will and masturbate in public.
  (5) <u>undifferentiated</u> - manifested by problems with reality testing, communications, thinking and interpersonal relationships.
- <u>Symptoms</u> may vary widely according to the severity and type of schizophrenia. The classical four symptoms are: ambivalence, associative disturbance, autism and affect impairment. Symptoms are usually broken into 2 categories: <u>cognitive</u> (e.g. disturbances of language & thought, distortion

of body image, feelings of depersonalization, hallucinations, delusions) and motor (e.g. withdrawal and isolation from others, inefficiency in performance). As a result of this symptomatology, the person focuses his interest and attention mainly on himself with resultant loss of social interaction, friendships, goal-oriented behavior. In severe disturbances, the patient becomes autistic and retreats into his world. The hospitalized schizophrenic is usually too disorganized and inefficient to maintain a job or school, to manage a home or his own affairs.

- Common behaviors include:
  1) withdrawal - people and events lose their meaning; the schizophrenic become indifferent to everything outside himself; he has no interest in other people or events; not in touch with reality enough to make goals.
  2) apathy with a flat (emotionless) affect - emotions seem to be minimal or absent; feelings may be out of keeping with the event.
  3) associative looseness - the schizophrenic's strange way of thinking and handling words makes it almost impossible for the observer to follow and understand what he is saying because the associations do not follow any logical sequence. This looseness with words is caused by autistic thinking; this thinking is so subjective and private that only the patient is aware of its meaning, and is an extreme retreat into fantasy.
  4) ambivalence - contradictory feelings of love, hate, fear which manifest in contradictory statements about a person or situation, or in the patient's inability to make decisions or express emotions. Ambivalence is a normal feeling that is greatly exaggerated in schizophrenic patients.
  5) impairment of process of reality testing - as manifested by: a. hallucinations: an imaginary sense perception during which the patient sees, hears, smells, or tastes things in a distorted way; patient may report this or behavior may suggest imaginary perception. Behaviors in response to hallucinations include: gestures, stereotyped mannerisms, actions which seem odd such as speaking to an empty room as if someone was present, nodding head, tilting head to one side. b. illusions: misinterpretation of an actual sensory experience, manifested by patient's statement of behavior; c. delusions: false, fixed belief that cannot be corrected by logic; manifested in dialogue, especially when the patient is experiencing stress; d. depersonalization: a feeling of not being quite real; manifested by patient's statements indicating that his own body has a strange and unreal feeling or that he has problems distinguishing himself from others; e. ideas of reference: the patient feels he is the subject of a conversation between others, and may be symbolic of feelings of guilt, insecurity and alienation.
  6) loss of interest in personal grooming, manifested by wearing same clothes daily, wearing oldest clothes, no makeup, lack of grooming for hair, nails, skin.

- Treatment: medication is the most effective type of treatment. With the advent of anti-psychotic drugs, many schizophrenic patients have been discharged from the hospital and are maintained in the community. Adherence to the prescribed medications is very important, as psychotic symptoms tend to reappear with a cutback in drugs. (See NCPG #3:45 "Drugs: Psychotropic") Other forms of treatment include group, individual, occupational, recreational and industrial therapy.

- Nursing responsibilities include interpreting and reinforcing reality to the patient, assisting him to manage his own life efficiently, supporting him in setting up goals for himself, and helping him to achieve some level of independence.

NCP Guide No. **3:37** 89

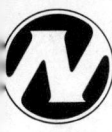

The Patient with <u>Schizophrenia</u>

Specific Considerations, Potential Patient Outcome and Nursing Actions:

1) Withdrawal Patient will learn to tolerate nurse's closeness and interest; patient will withdraw fewer times from contact with other persons:
- establish dialogue in order to be able to spend time, talk & plan with pt.; demonstrate an accepting attitude;
- plan with pt. convenient times to spend together; include 1-to-1 times as well as ward activities; listen & observe for non-verbal behaviors;
- use silence; share with pt. that you are willing to spend time without talking if he so chooses;
- observe pt's. pattern of social interaction and attendance at ward activities;
- support pt. with words & with your presence during activities which he finds frightening or difficult;
- discuss with pt. alternate ways to spend his day; describe his behaviors in a non-threatening way & indicate that you realize his difficulties in coping with the milieu;
- as pt. improves, provide anticipatory guidance for discharge; e.g. if pt. is experiencing withdrawal from social situations, role play the situation; encourage pt. to explore & pursue social situations where he feels most comfortable.

2) Apathetic with Flat Affect Patient will learn to identify feelings of anger, sadness, despair, loneliness; patient will share feelings with a staff or family member or another patient:
- observe pt.'s verbal & non-verbal expressions of feelings; share your observations with him in a non-judgmental way, e.g.—"This is what I notice and I'm wondering what you're feeling right now?" <u>or,</u> "You don't look to be upset right now, but if someone spit at me, I'd be mad." (or other behavior of another pt.);
- explore pt.'s feelings with him, accepting his right to feel as he does, no matter how illogical the feelings seem to you;
- give positive reinforcement for any expression of feeling and stay with pt. during this time;
- work with pt. to explore new ways to express feelings, e.g. to express anger, try handball, racketball, hitting a punching bag or bed, shouting, singing, confronting with words, swearing, batacus, tearing up phone books, throwing sponges or bean bags;
- expect exaggeration of expression combined with uncomfortable feelings when practicing this new behavior of expressing feelings;
- plan with pt. alternate ways to use feelings both within hospital and after discharge;
- observe verbal & non-verbal behaviors which may indicate any interest in activities; give support to any expression of interest;

- work with family/significant other to continue facilitation of pt.'s expression of feelings after discharge.

3) Associative Looseness — Patient will initiate conversation with staff or other patients; patient will learn to make his thinking understandable to others:
- listen to & chart patterns & symbols used in verbal communication; validate meaning with pt. before making an interpretation;
- look for patterns or themes in the pt.'s verbalization, i.e., "lovely princess in a tower; the dragons are trying to get me; I'm hooked up to all the TV stations and they control me…"
- be aware that pt.'s conversation can be filled with both rational and psychotic statements, out of sequence; define for the pt. those statements that are confusing to you, as a way to help keep him on the subject and facilitate communication and understanding;
- if pt. is having disassociated thoughts, talk about concrete realities, e.g., ward environment, his eating, sleeping & how he is feeling in the hospital;
- assign a permanent staff member to spend time each day interacting with & listening to the pt.; discuss goals & alternatives with him but avoid giving advice;
- discuss with pt. how his behavior affects and is viewed by others; point out, in a non-threatening way, how inappropriate behavior may alienate others.

4) Ambivalence — Patient will express and accept own ambivalent feelings:
- observe pt. for ambivalent feelings & attitudes; validate your observations, e.g., "Sometimes you hate your roommate & sometimes you love her; that's how you feel."
- discuss ambivalency as a normal state of being in all persons, which doesn't have to immobilize; accept pt.'s feelings of confusion or immobilization while continuing to work towards acceptance.

5) Impairment of Process of Reality Testing (Hallucination, Delusions, Ideas of Reference, Illusions) — Patient will learn to define and test reality; patient will learn to control impulsive behavior dictated by hallucinations and will dismiss the internal voices he hears:
- observe pt. for behavior indicating he is hearing voices (e.g. nodding head, or tilting it to one side, talking to people who are not present); when this occurs, ask pt. what is going on at this time (if you ask him if he is hearing voices, he is apt to say "no"); if he is hearing voices, discuss what hearing voices does for him, i.e., takes him away from painful/frustrating reality of interchange & relationships with others ("Right now, you'd rather listen to the voices than talk with Mr.—(or your wife, etc.)); help him focus on things in the immediate environment; do not give status or recognition to the voices;
- ask pt. if he has control over the voices; if not, supply controls with 1-to-1 support, or meds. (controls will make pt. feel more secure);
- know that pt. must dismiss the voices himself, and that he may be very anxious after this; when this occurs, alert staff so that all of you can provide extra support as temporary replacements for the voices;

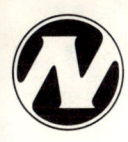

The Patient with <u>Schizophrenia</u>

- when pt. is hallucinating, have him name the fact that he is anxious and connect his behavior with it;
- if pt. is experiencing hallucinations, illusions, delusions, ideas of reference, interpret reality by telling him that you do not see or hear or believe these things, and that he must be feeling very anxious right now; do not talk to him about his delusions as that is non-therapeutic and pt. may become more out of control; rather, provide limits with a quiet room, walking or talking with pt. & meds; explore the basis for his feeling he is the subject of other conversations, and explain the reality of the actual situation to him;
- deal with & support reality: tell pt. your name, remind him where he is; be clear & concrete in your statements; look for reality stimuli that cause this stress & explore them with him;
- listen carefully to pt.; tell him when you do & do not understand;
- respond to the pt.'s thought disturbance, keeping in mind that the pt. is experiencing feelings of being overwhelmed; look for the reality stimuli causing the stress: e.g., a visit from a family member might trigger a thought disturbance, and explore possibilities with pt.;
- look for & chart behaviors, environmental stimuli that precipitate and/or relate to pt. withdrawing into fantasy; (when reality is too threatening, fantasy provides a comfortable retreat which will lower anxiety); accept pt.'s need for fantasy without supporting the context of it.

6) Loss of Interest in Taking Care of Self, in Personal Grooming, and Self-image

Patient will maintain good personal hygiene; patient will learn to manage own life in terms of personal grooming, taking medications; patient will strengthen interpersonal relationships:
- ensure that pt. bathes or showers at least Q1-2 days, dresses each day, and that he keeps own clothes clean; have him use washer-dryer PRN;
- provide an opportunity for pt. to groom nails & hair, & clean teeth; work with him to find an acceptable time & place for grooming activities;
- give positive reinforcement for good grooming and dress;
- observe & chart diet actually consumed; assess learning needs for balanced diet & teach PRN; use creative ways to encourage pt. to maintain adequate diet (juice, peanuts, milkshakes, cookie baking sessions, etc.);
- teach pt. the importance of taking his meds. daily; discuss their effect on him; as pt. improves, shift the responsibility of getting & taking meds to him, as preparation for discharge;

- observe physical condition & report problems to Dr.;
- plan with pt. ways he will maintain himself after discharge: e.g., caring for clothing, transportation, food shopping & meal preparation, recreation & work/school; help him set personal goals and support him in these;
- provide daily outlets for productive activity, e.g., occupational or industrial therapy; give positive rewards for all efforts; ask him what he would like to achieve, and help him with this goal;
- as discharge nears, discuss with pt. a follow-up care schedule, and develop a plan to use in case he feels depressed, out of touch with reality, spaced out, etc.;
- assess availability of significant others; include them in discharge planning, if possible.

Discharge Planning and Teaching Objectives/Outcomes:
1) (Patient and/or family/significant other) Has a list and schedule of medications, can verbalize the importance of taking them as prescribed, knows potential side effects, and knows how to obtain refills.
2) Has an appointment for follow-up care with Dr., clinic or day care center, etc., and knows to contact them if he feels a need before the appointment date.
3) Has a plan to maintain himself on a daily basis, that includes eating an adequate diet, maintaining personal grooming and interacting with others.
4) Knows importance of expressing feelings to others in order to facilitate communication and understanding, and to receive support during difficult times
5) Family/significant others are aware that patient often has difficulty expressing his feelings, and have learned to work with him to facilitate understanding.

Recommended References
"A Way to Communicate," by Alice D. Burkett, <u>American Journal of Nursing</u>, December 1974: 2185-2187.
"Biochemical Aspects of Schizophrenia," by Barbara M. Stewart, <u>American Journal of Nursing</u>, December 1975: 2176-2179.
"Disturbance in Language and Thought," by L. Crouch, <u>Journal of Psychiatric Nursing</u>, March-April 1972: 5-9.
"Drugs: Psychotropic," NCP Guide #3:46.
"Hallucinations and How to Deal with Them," by W. E. Field and W. Ruelke, <u>American Journal of Nursing</u>, April 1973: 638-640.
<u>I Never Promised You a Rose Garden</u>, by Hannah Green, New York: Holt, Rinehart & Winston, 1964.
<u>Psychiatric Nursing in the Hospital and Community</u>, by Burgess and Lazare, 2nd Ed., Englewood Cliffs, N.J.: Prentice-Hall, Inc., 1976.
"Recent Trends in Psychosocial Treatment of Schizophrenia," by L. R. Mosher, <u>American Journal of Psychoanalysis</u>, September 15, 1972: 9-15.
"Working with Schizophrenic Patients," —a special section, <u>American Journal of Nursing</u>, June 1976: 941-949.

© Margo Creighton Neal, 1977

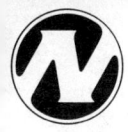

The Patient Experiencing Sensory Disturbances

Definition: A change in perception, level or type of response of an individual due to increased, decreased or absence of stimulation of the senses.

LONG TERM GOAL: The patient will regain and maintain sensory equilibrium.

General Considerations:
- **Sensory disturbances** occur in all acute care settings. With the advent of critical care units, life saving equipment, protective environments, and medical and nursing specialization, the intrusion on a person's environment, and/or lack of stimuli has increased and even contributed to morbidity rates.
- **Nursing assessment** focuses on observation of behavioral manifestations which include: (1) illusions, hallucinations and/or delusions, (2) withdrawal, (3) hostility (verbal attacks on staff), (4) crying or inappropriate affect, (5) confusion/disorientation of time, place, person, (6) sensory distortions e.g., incorrect perceptions of smell, touch, sight or response to treatment, (7) restlessness, (8) demand for constant reassurance about environment and treatment.
- **Nursing responsibilities** include an awareness of the *causes of sensory disturbances* to one or all senses (touch, smell, visualization and hearing). These causes include: (1) confinement in a small room; (2) lack of or excessive touching; (3) no verbal input or too much verbalization around the patient; (4) confinement in a windowless room; (5) discussion of hospital matters and/or information about other patients (these cause fear in addition to misperception of information related to the patient himself.); (6) continuous external stimuli, e.g., lights, monitors, staff/visitor verbalization; (7) lack of new stimuli; (8) placement in isolation; (9) change in external environment, e.g., new room, change in placement of equipment, personal supplies; (10) semi-consciousness and/or movement through different levels of consciousness causing a distortion (misperception) of what is heard, felt, seen or touched; and (11) separation from significant others. Interventions should focus on providing a stable environment for the patient by increasing or decreasing stimuli as needed.

Specific Considerations, Potential Patient Outcomes, and Nursing Actions:

1) Immediate Response to Recognition of Sensory Disturbance

The patient will be able to perceive and describe the components of his environment in an oriented, non-disturbed manner:
— talk directly to the pt.; make eye contact;
— use touch: give back rubs, massages, change position, stroke hair, etc.;
— give the pt. frequent, intermittent attention; do not isolate the pt. physically or emotionally; speak to the pt. each time you enter or leave the room;
— be aware of environmental monotony; use clocks, calendars, pictures, pt.'s personal possessions to stimulate & encourage pt. to explore his surroundings;

- give the pt. several periods of rest intermixed with stimulation throughout the day, rather than continuous stimulation;
- reduce or eliminate staff discussions of pts., hospital and/or personal matters in and around any pt.'s room or bed;
- identify what you are going to do each time you see the pt.; consider & utilize safety precautions as needed;
- some disturbances are caused by recumbent position alone; provide opportunities to sit, stand or be partially upright; give passive or active exercises;
- confusion that is physiological in nature cannot be controlled by behavioral approaches; however, it is important to approach the pt. often & give kind reassurances; do not increase fear & confusion by avoiding the pt.

2) Restoration to Adaptive Coping

The patient will be able to identify stimuli which are conducive to his treatment and recovery and stimuli which increase fear, anxiety, and restlessness:
- plan the care & daily activities with the pt.; evaluate the nursing care with the pt.;
- blind and/or deaf pts. have special needs due to the lack of these senses; make sure that these pts. have the opportunity to express these needs & have them met; communicate to all staff the sensory facilities the pt. may be lacking; e.g. blind, or without his glasses; deaf & without a hearing aid;
- ask the pt. to tell you when the stimuli is too little or too much . . . e.g., "It's so noisy." "I would like to rest." Attempt to reduce or increase the stimuli to meet the pt.'s needs;
- control levels of light, noise, odors, sights to tolerable levels; provide change of scenery, walks, rides, conversations with other pts., recreational or occupational therapy, & social activities as appropriate;
- have staff observe how the pt. is responding to them & the care they are giving (remember, the pt.'s response is a mirror of his need, not a response you take personally);
- make sure that all staff & significant others are aware of the pt.'s need for intermittent rest & stimulation; sensory overload mixed with deprivation does not allow the pt. to cope adequately with the hospitalization;
- provide the pt. with stimuli in the form of conversation, playing games, reading to him;
- refer pts. with long-term sensory impairments to the appropriate community resources, e.g. Society for the Blind.

Discharge Planning and Teaching Objectives/Outcomes
1) (Patient/Family/Significant Other) Can identify external environmental stimuli which are necessary for daily functioning.
2) Can identify external stimuli which cause fear, anxiety and reduce his ability to function.
3) Can identify and utilize sources of support to deal with sensory overload and/or deprivation situations.

Recommended References

"Bedrest and Sensory Disturbances." by Florence Downs. *American Journal of Nursing*, March 1974:434–438.

"Communication in the ICU: Therapeutic or Disturbing," by Mary Anne Noble. *Nursing Outlook*, March 1979:195–198.

"Sensory Alterations. Overload and Underload: Making a Nursing Diagnosis," by Mary Jane Barry, in M. Kennedy and G. Pfeifer, *Volume One: Current Practice in Nursing Care of the Adult—Issues and Concepts*. St. Louis: C.V. Mosby Co., 1979:33–45.

The Patient Experiencing Shame/Embarrassment

Definition: Shame is a subjective feeling of a sudden sense of painful self-consciousness and embarrassment, ranging from mild to intense humiliation.

LONG TERM GOAL: The patient will share feelings of shame and will participate in problem solving to avoid and manage these feelings.

General Considerations:
— Shame may be evoked by situations in which the patient experiences actual or potential loss of control or function and by invasion of body boundaries or territory; incontinence of urine or bowel movement is threatening. Shame may be experienced during admission procedures, when dressing or undressing, bathing, during examinations or treatments, while sharing a room with a stranger, or when experiencing intense feelings or pain.
— Shame can be perceived as an important self-message of conflict of values and behavior; it can provide an opportunity to: 1) increase self-awareness of attitudes and feelings, and 2) to learn alternative coping methods.
— **Characteristic behaviors** include:
  - blushing or blanching of face, neck and chest
  - avoiding eye contact, lowering eyes, blinking
  - turning face away/covering face with hands
  - hand to mouth movement
  - change in voice and speech pattern
  - twisting fingers or hands
  - nervous adjustment of hair or clothes
  - shuffling feet
  - embarrassed laugh
  - tremor in hands
  - exaggerated "chin up" (anti-shame posture)
  - patient describes feelings of embarrassment or shame
  - patient uses negative labeling of self, i.e., "I'm such a baby." "I'm dirty," "I'm dumb," "I'm disgusting."
— **Nursing responsibilities** include anticipating and preventing situations which could evoke shame or embarrassment, recognizing shame/embarrassment behaviors, intervening immediately to alleviate distress, and teaching alternative coping methods.

Specific Considerations, Potential Patient Outcomes, and Nursing Actions:

1) Prevention of Shame/Embarrassment — The patient will maintain self-respect and dignity:
   — maintain respectful & courteous relationship with pt. & family; call pt. by name, knock on door, provide privacy;
   — encourage individuality & respect differences; assess individual preferences & note on care plan;
   — explain all procedures & hospital routines; provide as much information as you think pt. wants & needs;
   — encourage pt. to anticipate new situations & explore concerns & questions;

		— role-play potential situations & develop new responses;
		— spend time with pt. listening to concerns, assisting pt. with ADL, & building a trust relationship;
		— know that most feelings of shame can be prevented.
2)	Immediate Response to Recognition of Shame	The patient will acknowledge shame/embarrassment and maintain self-respect: — assess for non-verbal & verbal shame behaviors; — assess pt.'s perception of self & situation; — encourage pt. to acknowledge feelings to one other person; — accept pt.'s feelings & validate him as a unique person; — explore shame situation: in what way does the pt. feel embarrassed? humiliated? — determine if hospital procedures or staff behaviors caused pt. to experience shame; if so, make amends & manage environment to prevent causes.
3)	Alternative Coping Methods	The patient will develop new ways of coping with situations which evoke shame or embarrassment: — assess pt.'s attitudes towards self & expectations of self in situation; — teach pt. that shame/embarrassment is common & normal & often can be anticipated & prevented; — explore "shoulds," i.e., what the pt. thinks s/he should do; support realistic expectations & correct unrealistic ones (e.g., pt. may not know expected behaviors for sick role & may feel shame at being dependent on others, sharing a bedroom with other people, exposing body for examinations, or experiencing intense feelings of fear or loss, grief & mourning); — assess for lack of experience or skills in communication, assertiveness, or interpersonal relationships; pt. may not know how to ask for privacy or how to negotiate for special needs or wants; health teach using problem solving, behavior modification, & practice of desired behaviors (see NCPG #5:47, "Problem Solving," #5:38, "Behavior Modification," and #1:49, "Teaching Patient."); — problem solve with pt. to restore self-respect & to avoid or change situation which evoked the shame.

Recommended References

"Behavior Modification." *NCP Guide #5:37*, Nurseco, 1981.
"The Effect of Hospitalization on Guilt and Shame Feelings," by Ilhan M. Ermutlu. *Psychiatric Forum*, Winter 1977:18–23.
"Problem Solving." *NCP Guide #5:47*, Nurseco, 1981.
"Shame," by Silvia Lange. *Behavioral Concepts and Nursing Interventions*, C. Carlson & B. Blackwell, Eds. Philadelphia: J.B. Lippincott Co., 1978:51–71.
"Stress Management." *NCP Guide #5:49*, Nurseco, 1981.
"Teaching Patients: General Suggestions." *NCP Guide #1:49*, 2nd Ed., Nurseco, 1980.

NCP Guide No. **1:33** ·97

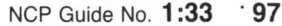

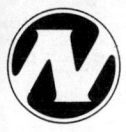

The Patient Experiencing Shock, Psychogenic

Definition: A state in which a person tries to insulate or protect self from a major event or imagined danger which is too much to handle all at once.

LONG TERM GOAL: The patient will be able to discuss the traumatic event and share positive and negative aspects of it.

General Considerations:
- **Psychogenic shock** is a response to a traumatic (real or imagined) event that confronts the individual. The person does not expect the event and cannot cope with the reality of it.
- **Nursing assessment** includes awareness of the manifestations of psychogenic shock which include:
  - silence;
  - crying;
  - denial of the causative event;
  - uncooperative manner;
  - unresponsiveness, appearing stunned or dazed;
  - apathetic, acting as if devoid of feeling;
  - unable to concentrate, to understand explanations and/or retain information;
  - feelings of helplessness, hopelessness or abandonment;
  - aimless wandering or puttering at small tasks;
  - hostility and/or blaming staff for the causative event.
- **Nursing responsibilities** include monitoring the patient's responses and activities since the patient is generally unable to cope without outside support.
- **Nursing interventions** should be directed toward allowing the patient time to come to grips with the situation and perceive the reality of it.

Specific Considerations, Potential Patient Outcomes, and Nursing Actions:

1) Immediate Response to Recognition of Psychogenic Shock

The patient will be able to allow others to assist him to cope:
- remain with the pt. for at least fifteen minutes or until replaced by another caring person;
- some denial of the event is important & necessary, but encourage the growing acceptance of reality;
- allow & encourage coping mechanisms such as crying, silence, walking, reliving the event;
- listen sympathetically, sharing the experience as the pt. permits you to do so.

2) Restoration to Adaptive Coping

The patient will return to responsiveness and responsible activity; will have a continuing human resource who will be helpful In a healthy way:
— assess what needs to be done & provide only the help that is really necessary;
— explore problem-solving options with the pt., but permit him to make his own decisions if they can be reality-based;
— allow the pt. to do as much as s/he can, but have another supportive person handle frustrating, complicated details & complex activities for the present;
— explain to the "supportive other" what the pt. is going through, how s/he is progressing, that the behavior is normal under the circumstances, & what can be expected of the pt. as s/he recovers from this state of shock (e.g. nightmares, possible physical complaints, resentment of others);
— verbally reward the "helper" for his interest, concern & willingness to be involved & available to the pt.;
— help this person to realize the pt.'s need to regain control of own life, to make decisions, & to do for self as much as possible;
— ask the "helping person" to use own personality strengths, i.e., warmth, humor, listening skill, etc., to sustain the pt. in moments of fleeting sadness, guilt, fear, etc.

Discharge Planning and Teaching Objectives/Outcomes
1) (Patient/Family/Significant Other) Can acknowledge the existence of the traumatic event.
2) Can allow others to be physically and emotionally supportive as needed.
3) Can demonstrate the ability to provide for own food, clothing and shelter.

Recommended References
"Grief and Grieving," by George Engel. *American Journal of Nursing*, September 1965:93.
"Helping Survivors Cope with the Shock of Sudden Death," by Patricia Sharer. *Nursing 79*, January 1979:20–23.
"Responses to Loss." *NCP Guide* #1:31, 2nd Ed., Nurseco, 1980.
"Sharing a Tragedy," by Judith Breuer. *American Journal of Nursing*, May 1976:758–759.
"Solving the Riddle of Loss:'Depression' and other Responses." Filmstrips available from Nurseco, PO Box 145, Pacific Palisades, CA 90272.
"The Simple Act of Touching," by James J. Lynch. *Nursing 78*, June 1978:32–36.

© Margo Creighton Neal, 1980

The Patient Adapting to the Sick Role

Definition: The sick role consists of the behaviors that are defined by society as appropriate to the patient's stage of illness and position on the health-illness continuum.

LONG TERM GOAL: The patient will adapt to the sick role by taking on behaviors appropriate to the current stage of illness and convalescence.

General Considerations:
- **Socialization** is a dynamic, lifelong process in which the individual acquires attitudes and values, assumes new and different roles, and learns the behaviors and skills that go with the roles.
- **Role learning and role change** take place mainly in daily interpersonal relationships. Individuals usually have several roles simultaneously including family, work, and social roles.
- There are three stages of role change in the cycle of health and illness: transition from health to illness, the period of actual illness, and convalescence.
- **Nursing responsibilities** include assessing the patient for behavioral manifestations of adaptive or maladaptive sick role, and prescribing interventions to facilitate adaptive sick role and convalescence or treat maladaptive sick role.
- **Characteristic behaviors:**

ADAPTIVE SICK ROLE	MALADAPTIVE SICK ROLE
Stage I, Transition from Health to Illness	
Recognizes symptoms; may have some shock and disbelief.	Does not recognize symptoms or completely denies symptoms.
Seeks care of health care worker or doctor.	Does not seek care of health care provider or doctor.
Tells of symptoms, problems, concerns.	Makes no mention of symptoms, problems, concerns, or exaggerates or confuses them; quiet or hyperactive.
Stage II, Actual Illness	
Participates with health care worker to plan treatment, set priorities.	Refuses to participate in treatment plan.
Complies with treatment plan.	Does not comply with treatment plan; unresponsive or negative.
Seeks relief from usual roles and responsibilities.	Continues with usual roles and responsibilities inappropriately.
Asks for aid from spouse, friends, family.	Does not request aid; does everything or nothing.
Asks for acceptance of illness and love in spite of illness.	Defensive or aggressive, passive-aggressive behaviors; may be seductive toward staff.
Talks about body functions and progress; preoccupied with	Complains constantly and does not acknowledge progress;

self and somatic concerns.
Shares feelings and concerns; ambivalent with dependency; both grateful and resentful.
Asks for help appropriately from staff.

Stage III, Convalescence
Asks for guidance in resuming previous roles and responsibilities.

Asks for help from spouse, friends, family, and co-workers in resuming previous tasks.
Anticipates needs and asks for convalescent medication, treatment, activity, and rest orders.
Convalesces and returns to previous state of health.

negative or denies concerns or problems.
Does not express or seem aware of own feelings.

Asks for care from others which s/he is capable of doing for self, or will not ask for help; demands, withdraws, complains constantly.

Does not ask for guidance; assumes roles and responsibilities prematurely or not at all.
Does not ask for help; does too much, too little for self; resents offers of help.
Does not think ahead and refuses to discuss treatment plan for convalescence.
Refuses to give up sick role; perceives self as sick when care givers perceive as convalescent or healthy.

Specific Considerations, Potential Patient Outcomes, and Nursing Actions:

1) Stage I, Transition from Health to Illness

The patient moves adaptively from health to illness by recognizing and reporting symptoms and by seeking care of health worker:
— establish self as a concerned & helpful professional who wants to understand pt. & family & their concerns; encourage the pt. to describe symptoms & share feelings, concerns;
— orient the pt. & family to immediate environment; answer questions;
— assess pt.'s knowledge of procedures & health teach as needed, giving descriptions with simple, non-tension producing words; include what the pt. will feel, hear, see, taste, experience;
— assess pt. & family for behaviors of anxiety & fear; these may include excessive demands, refusal to cooperate, withdrawal, not asking questions; see NCPGs #1:22, "The Patient Experiencing Anxiety" & #1:28, "The Patient Experiencing Fear;"
— assess pt. for behaviors of shock & disbelief, denial, & other behaviors of loss; listen & give emotional support, accepting

the pt.'s need to cope with the situation at his own pace; see NCPGs #1:24, "The Patient Manifesting Denial" & #1:31, "Responses to Loss: The Grief and Mourning Process."

2) Stage II, Actual Illness

The patient adapts to sick role by participating in setting goals and planning care; the patient cooperates with the treatment plan:
— assess pt. & family goals, priorities, & preferences; include these in care plan; work with pt. to set goals & plan care; offer support & information as needed;
— discuss concerns pt. may have with letting go of usual family, work, or social roles & responsibilities; encourage pt. to ask for help from spouse, family, & friends;
— encourage pt. to ventilate feelings & concerns about illness, hospitalization, body functions, progress, prognosis; accept feelings & preoccupation with somatic concerns;
— assess pt.'s knowledge of diet, medications, treatments, activity, rest, & diagnosis; health teach as needed;
— encourage pt. to do appropriate self-care; offer emotional support & praise; see NCPG #5:37, "Behavior Modification;"
— be aware that pt. may have lost independence & self-esteem as a result of illness & hospitalization; accept ambivalent feelings of gratitude & resentment towards staff, family, friends.

3) Stage III, Convalescence

The patient makes transition from illness to convalescence by participation in and cooperation with convalescent treatment plan:
— discuss progress & anticipate convalescence with pt. & family;
— assist pt. to resume roles & responsibilities as appropriate; encourage pt. to ask for help from staff, spouse, friends, family, co-workers;
— using anticipatory guidance, assist pt. to plan for discharge from hospital; problem solve & health teach as needed to be sure pt. & family understand discharge orders such as medication, treatments, activity, rest, diet, when to call physician; see NCPG #5:47, "Problem Solving;"
— assist pt. & family to explore community resources such as VNA, "Meals on Wheels," hospital equipment rental, homemaker service, Cancer Society, Colostomy Club (or other self-help groups);
— ask open-ended questions such as, "How do you plan to manage . . . ? "What are your plans for . . . ?"

Discharge Planning and Teaching Objectives/Outcomes
1) (Patient/Family/Significant Other) Can recognize appropriate behaviors in illness and convalescence.
2) Can describe plan for adapting to possible future sick role.

Recommended References
"Behavior Modification." *NCP Guide #5:37*, Nurseco, 1981.
"The Effects of Hospitalization: Part A: Tension Producing Causes." *NCP Guide #1:40*, 2nd Ed., Nurseco, 1980.
"The Effects of Hospitalization: Part B: Assessment." *NCP Guide #1:41*, 2nd Ed., Nurseco, 1980.
"The Effects of Hospitalization: Part C: Prolonged Confinement." *NCP Guide #1:42*, 2nd Ed., Nurseco, 1980.
"The Patient Experiencing Anxiety." *NCP Guide #1:22*, 2nd Ed., Nurseco, 1980.
"The Patient Experiencing Fear." *NCP Guide #1:28*, 2nd Ed., Nurseco, 1980.
"The Patient Manifesting Denial." *NCP Guide #1:24*, 2nd Ed., Nurseco, 1980.
"Problem Solving." *NCP Guide #5:47*, Nurseco, 1981.
"Responses to Loss: The Grief and Mourning Process." *NCP Guide #1:31*, 2nd Ed., Nurseco, 1980.
"Symptom Reports and Illness Behavior Among Employed Women and Homemakers," by N.F. Woods et al. *Journal of Community Health*, Fall 1979:36–45.

NCP Guide No. **3:38** 103

The Patient who is <u>Suicidal</u> (on a Psychiatric Unit)

LONG TERM GOAL: The patient will be free of suicidal ideation, thoughts and feelings, and will develop new alternatives to cope with the conditions which contributed to the suicidal state.

General Considerations:

- Suicide <u>may be defined</u> as an act to voluntarily end one's own life; it may be the ultimate act of self-hatred, or an attempt to control the time and circumstances of death. Suicide is a method of communication, a "cry for help," a visible sign that the person wishes to escape an intolerable situation and has run out of positive alternatives.
- <u>Statistics:</u> suicide has ranked among the 12 leading causes of death in the U.S. for several years; it is the 3rd leading cause of death in the 15-19 year old age group. and the 2nd leading cause of death on college campuses, with the rate for men twice as high as for women. In 1974, more than 25,000 suicides were recorded; it is believed that a more accurate figure would be 2-3 times greater.
- <u>Population at risk</u>: Suicide is higher in single, widowed, separated and divorced people. In the U.S., it is more prevalent in white than non-white persons; also high for migrants, foreign-born, the aged and those living alone; is associated with alcoholism and homicide. Suicide in the aged is associated with physical and mental illness, social isolation, death of a loved one, loss of income or status (especially in retirement). Danger points for suicide are stressful situational or maturational events or passage through the usual developmental phases. (Read NCPG's #2:31 & 2:35, "Crisis Intervention.")
- <u>Family patterns of young people who commit suicide</u> often include parents who strive overtly for success for themselves and their children, who see their children as extensions of their fantasized successes and block out other kinds of communication, especially those implying failure by their children. These parental expectations are far more intense than the usual wishes for success that parents have for children; they represent a total lack of acceptance of their children the way they are. Most young people who attempt suicide feel that their family doesn't accept or understand them; they are reported to have had physical fights with family members and have family histories of physical and assaultive behaviors in family members. These same factors that make them unhappy enough to commit suicide often lead to alcohol and drug use.
- <u>Common behaviors</u> include: nagging lack of optimism and hope about future, intense sense of unhappiness, depression and inability to control own impulses; agitation and restlessness, which may increase as the person experiences loss of impulse control; loss of impulse control in some people may be accompanied by withdrawal, apathy and immobility; helplessness and dependency; social isolation (few contacts with neighbors, family or friends); intense loneliness (a subjective feeling unrelated to social isolation); marked hostility and anger.

- Warnings (or clues): Studies show that suicidal persons give many verbal and/or non-verbal warnings or clues of suicidal plans, e.g. giving things away that they usually need, making a will, checking on life insurance; pointed questions such as, "How do you go about giving your body to science? Does this hospital use kidneys or eyes donated before a person dies?" or statements concerning thoughts of death... "If I died, I'd want a white casket and white flowers," or even: "Goodbye, nurse," (which can be a significant statement if the timing or wording is different from usual.) Statements such as "I'm too far gone for anyone to help me," or "The world's a jungle and I can't face it," give clues to the person's hopelessness and helplessness.
- A psychiatric diagnosis is one of the key prognostic factors in assessing the risk of suicide attempt to repeating suicide attempt. Frequently encountered diagnoses will be:
  - Depression: Patient may state "I deserve to be dead,"... "My wife and children are better off without me,"... "I just can't face it anymore." There is increased risk as an out-patient if: (a) depressive symptoms are severe with marked change in ability to care for self or marked feelings of hopelessness or guilt; (b) extremely agitated and impulsive; (c) out of contact with reality; or (d) pattern of continuing suicidal ideation.
  - Schizophrenia: High suicidal risk if patient is experiencing delusions or hallucinations; may include hostile voices which tell him to injure self.
  - Organic brain syndrome: suicidal risk is increased if patient is repeating negative or self-defeating patterns, deals with stress by use of alcohol or drugs, demonstrates impulsive behavior, has limited adaptive responses, has mood swings, is confused or indicates may have delusions, illusions, or hallucinations.
  - Personality disorders: (1) hysterical personality—includes dependent behaviors and acting out; suicide often a gesture or power play. (2) chronic alcoholic—demanding, dependent behavior with disordered interpersonal relationships. Solves problems with alcohol which increases vulnerability to negative and impulsive behaviors. (3) antisocial personality—impulsive, demanding and manipulative in egocentric way; has history of behavior harmful to others. Suicide may be manipulation of social situation. May be threat to self and others.
- Treatment aims include decreasing the overwhelming feelings of helplessness and hopelessness, increasing impulse control and developing positive alternatives.
- Nursing Responsibilities include: prevention (by recognition of behaviors of persons at risk), assessment of lethality of intent, and working with patient/client to restore hope and develop positive alternatives. It also includes providing self and other staff with a supportive environment, since working with suicidal patients is emotionally draining and anxiety-producing. (This supportive environment includes daily supervision and informal discussion regarding feelings about suicide, death, hostility, anger, depression and other painful emotions.) Developing an on-going relationship with a suicidal patient is an intense experience in which both persons in the relationship examine their existential feelings about the value of life and the meaning of life and death. It is an opportunity for the staff member to share her commitment to life, her hope and caring for the other person. If the staff member does not receive support and supervision, she will be unable to develop this kind of intense, caring relationship; both she and the patient will experience increased anxiety and will then have less energy to work towards hope and health.

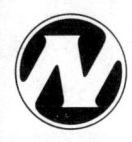

The Patient who is <u>Suicidal</u> (on a Psychiatric Unit)

Specific Considerations, Potential Patient Outcomes and Nursing Actions:

1) Observation & Protection; Helpful Relationships

The patient will be safe from injury; the patient will establish a trusting relationship and rapport with at least one staff member:
- assume responsibility for safety of pt. (a priority): inspect ward for potentially hazardous situations; make sure windows are shatter-proof or use first floor facilities; remove sharp objects such as scissors, nail files, razor blades, and medication from pt's. access (may be used only with 1-to-1 supervision);
- restrict pt. to observable areas of ward, deciding when he may leave unit with staff, visitors or alone; use 1-to-1 staffing as needed;
- plan staffing so that unit is always covered by experienced staff, especially at staff meal times, breaks, vacations, change of shift; suicide occurs most often in hospital settings during change of shift, at mealtimes, or on weekends;
- assess for suicide plan & lethality: when, where, how, with what tools; plans are <u>most lethal</u> when they are specific, i.e. person has planned specific time and isolated place, or plans severe or self-mutilating act such as large amount of lethal meds; <u>less lethal</u> when plans are vague or plans a minor dose of meds, or superficial cut wrist in a place where can be discovered;
- assess intensity of wish to die and determination; pt's. statements and affect are best indicators;
- assess past history: past unresolved losses, history of previous suicidal attempt in patient or pt's. family; (previous attempt increases risk); is pt. in therapy and is therapist available? (pt. is at risk if therapist is on vacation or unavailable);
- assess pt's. perception of situation and feeling about it and himself; listen for his level of hope, his view of the situation as being intolerable, his feelings of inadequacy in coping with present and past stresses, his loss or expected loss, his frustrations, feelings of unworthiness. <u>If pt. has attempted suicide,</u> listen for his attitude about the attempt; is he sorry he didn't succeed and threatening to try again; does he regret his behavior and plan to come for help if he feels that he is going out of control?
- assess social network: does pt. have a significant other, i.e. close friend or family member; is this person available?; is relationship under increased stress at this time or has there been a loss of this relationship? The more friends a person has, the stronger is his support system;
- assess current life situation: ask pt. to describe it to you; look for stress situation, intensity of stress, losses, increased depression, loss of hope;

NCP Guide No. **3:38 106**

- spend time with pt. to observe behaviors & begin building a trusting relationship; relationship & rapport with staff is one of most important deterrents to suicide; know that this pt. has an intense need to trust, to be accepted, to increase self-esteem; respect, caring & concern are vitally important to him.

2) Inability to Cope with Painful Feelings

The patient will identify and talk about painful feelings he is experiencing:
- see consideration #1 ("Inability to Cope with Painful Feelings") in NCPG #3:35, "Depression (Psychiatric)."

3) Inability to Perform Self-Care Activities

The patient will resume self-care in grooming; the patient will ingest adequate foods and fluids, and achieve an adequate sleep-rest-activity pattern:
- if pt. suffers from insomnia, assign a staff person to check on him @ 1/2 hr. intervals and spend time with him during night; early morning hours may be most difficult time for this patient, and the time when he needs a nurse's presence the most;
- see consideration #2 ("Inability to Perform Self-Care Activities") in NCPG #3:35, "Depression (Psychiatric)", eliminating #7 of that section.

4) Intense Loneliness; Difficulty with Social Relationships

The patient will experience less loneliness; the patient will show increased ability to make contact in social relationships:
- see consideration #4 ("Social Relationships") in NCPG #3:35, "Depression (Psychiatric)."

Discharge Planning and Teaching Objectives/Outcomes:
1) thru 4) Same as for "Depression (Psychiatric)", NCPG #3:35, plus:
5) (Family/significant other) Can identify high suicidal risk behaviors and has worked out a suitable crisis plan.

Recommended References
"Crisis Intervention," NCP Guide #2:35, NURSECO: 1975.
"The Patient Needing Crisis Intervention," NCP Guide #2:31, NURSECO: 1975.
"The Patient Experiencing Depression (Psychiatric)," NCP Guide #3:35.
"Suicide," by T. Westercamp, American Journal of Nursing, February, 1975: 260-262.
"Suicide: an Invitation to Die," by S. Jourard, American Journal of Nursing, February, 1970: 269.
"Suicide in Relation to Time of Day and Day of the Week," by K. Vollen and C. Watson, American Journal of Nursing, February, 1975: 263.

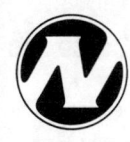

The Patient who has Attempted Suicide (admitted to a Med-Surg. Unit)

LONG TERM GOAL: The patient will recover from the suicidal attempt, and will establish a link to a mental health professional for continuing care.

General Considerations:
- Read NCPG's #3:38, "The Patient who is Suicidal" and #3:35, "The Patient Experiencing Depression."
- <u>Precipitating factors</u> in a suicidal crisis are usually a real or threatened loss (of a loved one, prestige, hope, job, money, health, body part, etc.) and the resultant overwhelming feelings of loneliness, depression, hopelessness and helplessness. Read NCPG #1:31, "Responses to Loss..." and NCPG's #2:31 and 2:35, "Crisis Intervention."
- <u>Many nurses and other staff on a med-surg. unit often experience anger and frustration</u> in caring for patients who have attempted suicide, especially with "repeaters." While nurses and staff are working hard to save lives, it is difficult for them to understand the painful feelings the patient is experiencing. Staff have a responsibility to recognize own feelings in regard to suicide and patients who have attempted, to share these with others and to give and receive support. Refer to "Nursing Responsibilities" in NCPG #3:38, "The Suicidal Patient."
- <u>Nursing Responsibilities</u> include: carrying out measures to maintain physiological homostasis, to provide non-judgmental care for the patient in a warm, caring manner and to try to understand the patient's feelings that led to the suicidal attempt. Persons who attempt suicide are usually overwhelmed with feelings of loneliness, hopelessness and not knowing where to turn. Empathic, caring nurses can begin to restore their hope.

Specific Considerations, Potential Patient Outcomes and Nursing Actions:

1) Restoration of Physiological Integrity

The patient will stabilize physiologically, free of preventable complications; the patient will recover from the suicide attempt in a safe, non-threatening and non-judgmental environment:
- maintain pt's life by measures dictated by his state of consciousness: e.g. keep airway patent with suctioning PRN, have pt. cough or use blow bottles & turn from side to side PRN, etc.;
- if pt. comatose, maintain Foley catheter, body alignment & skin integrity, with usual maintenance nursing measures; do neuro checks Q30 mins.;
- monitor vital signs @ least hourly; report changes to Dr.; record I&O, observing urinary output hourly, as an indication of renal function;
- if pt. has overdosed, determine, if possible, type & amount of drug taken and its expected side effects.

2) Overwhelming Painful Feelings

The patient will identify and talk about some of the painful feelings he is experiencing; the patient will verbalize his perceptions of his current situation; the patient will experience a lessening of anxiety and feelings of helplessness and hopelessness:
- openly admit your recognition of pt. as a troubled, unhappy person _and_ your willingness to listen - ("I am really concerned about you! I want to help."... "Things must have looked pretty hopeless to you.");
- listen to what the pt. says, allowing him to talk at length without challenging his statements; reinforce reality: do not support denial, but rather share how you see it: ("This is how I see, feel, hear it...");
- assess pt's. attitude re: failure of the suicide attempt and the nature of the intent - ("What did you hope would happen when you took the pills? What do you hope will happen now?"); discuss positive alternatives that pt. could choose to change current situation; provide positive reinforcement at every opportunity;
- assess pt's. need for safety & assume this responsibility PRN: know your hospital's policy re: 1-to-1 staffing by staff or family/friends; know & reinforce to others that mandatory 1-to-1 staffing should focus on the pt. and the painful feelings he is experiencing with the goal of reducing them as noted above (this is often difficult for staff to do _unless_ they have worked through their own feelings re: suicide);
- review NCPG #3:38, "The Patient who is Suicidal" and #'s 2:31 & 2:35, "Crisis Intervention."

3) Discharge Planning

The patient will establish a professional mental health link to deal with the precipitating factors on a continuing basis:
- discuss with pt. his plans after discharge; does he see the need for mental health counseling/therapy? point out that such follow-up will enable him to deal with his situation in a much healthier & better way than he can probably do on his own;
- learn what the pt. is willing to do to help himself; will he talk to a clergyman, school counselor or teacher, social worker or psychiatric nurse, mental health specialist or psychologist, psychiatrist? discuss possible referrals with pt's. Dr., & with pt.; it is important to find a referral that is acceptable to pt.;
- initiate follow-up referrals to an appropriate community mental health clinic, psychiatric care facility, private psychiatrist, psychologist or certified psychiatric nurse.

Discharge Planning and Teaching Objectives/Outcomes:
1) (Patient and/or family/significant other) Knows that telephone assistance is always available at local Suicide Prevention Center, Hot Line or Help Line and has the telephone number(s).
2) Has a referral for follow-up mental health counseling/therapy.
3) Family is aware of some cries for help and knows to stay with patient at these times, and to seek professional help.

NCP Guide No. **3:39 109**

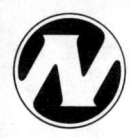

The Patient who has <u>Attempted Suicide</u> (admitted to a Med-Surg. Unit)

Recommended References
"Crisis Intervention," NCP Guide #2:35, NURSECO: 1975.
"The Patient Experiencing Depression (Psychiatric)," NCP Guide #3:35.
"The Patient Needing Crisis Intervention," NCP Guide #2:31, NURSECO: 1975.
"The Patient who is Suicidal (on a Psychiatric Unit)," NCP Guide #3:38.
"Responses to Loss: the Grief and Mourning Process," NCP Guide #1:31, NURSECO: 1974.
"Suicide," by T. Westercamp, <u>American Journal of Nursing</u>, February, 1975: 260-262.
"You Can Prevent Suicide," by M. O. Dinan, <u>Nursing '76</u>, January: 60-64.

©Margo Creighton Neal, 1977

NCP Guide No. **4:40** 111

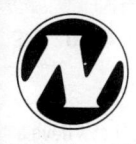

The Patient who is <u>Violent</u>

Definition: <u>Violence</u> is any physical behavior that is destructive to self, others or property.
<u>Acting out</u> is any aggressive/angry behavior short of violence and includes verbal and non-verbal threats.
<u>Aggression</u> is a state of inner tension causing some discomfort to an individual and energizing him to overcome his environment, often using gross motor behavior.

LONG TERM GOAL: The patient will develop new alternatives to deal with aggressive impulses.

General Considerations:
- <u>Principles and procedures</u> for control of aggression, acting out and violence should be a part of every mental health facility's routine inservice training, review procedure for your facility.
- A <u>therapeutic milieu</u> adequately staffed by well trained and caring health care workers can prevent most violence.
- <u>Each violent incident should be reviewed</u> with a goal of improving patient care by identifying situations which contribute to violence and by evaluating and revising interventions.
- <u>Interventions</u> which decrease perceived threat and diminish feelings of impotence in the patient are usually most successful. The theoretical reason for this is that violence is a response to feelings of impotence and helplessness in the face of a perceived threat. This threat may come at the time of admission to a mental health facility: the patient may feel that his worst fear has come true, for he has lost control of his behavior and is "crazy" and being locked up. This may be accompamied by a marked increase in anxiety behaviors as he realizes that he must obey the rules or take the consequences. With a threat from within and a threat from without, a patient may respond with fight, flight, or freeze responses. He is not allowed to leave the hospital; he may flee to his room, which he must share with other patients, and he feels increasingly impotent. As anxiety and stress increase, the ability to reason decreases, and the patient responds more to isolated stimuli and less to the content of the situation. See NCP Guides #1:20, "Aggression," and 1:21, "Anger" for interventions to prevent violence.

Specific Considerations, Potential Patient Outcomes and Nursing Actions:

1) Immediate Response to Violent Behavior

Patient will stop violent behavior:
- allow pt. to remain in present physical position; give pt. space & keep some distance away;
- observe pt. while placing self between pt. & door if possible; do not turn back to pt; move slowly & deliberately;
- ask other pts. to withdraw & leave area; speak in a calm, quiet tone;

- identify feeling of anxiety: "You seem upset; I'm concerned you might hurt yourself or others here;"
- encourage verbalization rather than acting out: "What happened to make you so upset just now?";
- offer alternatives: "I'll walk with you and we can talk about this." "Let's walk back to your room and discuss this." "Let's have a cup of coffee and talk about it." "I'll stay with you while you hit the punching bag.";
- provide reassurance of support and set limits: "I want to help you control your behavior right now so that you do not hurt yourself or someone else."

2) Increasing Violent Behavior; Physical Restraints

The patient will tolerate physical restraints to prevent expression of violence:
- assemble equipment & staff; 4 staff members necessary to restrain average sized pt.; if time available, staff should remove glasses or pens or other potentially harmful articles from their person; a blanket or sheet & soft leather arm & leg restraints may be needed;
- prepare a private room which contains a bed with a metal frame to which restraints can be secured; clear this room of other potentially dangerous items; hallway to room should be cleared of pts. & visitors;
- explain to pt.: "We're concerned about this behavior and we're going to help you control it now so that you don't hurt yourself or others;"
- distract the pt. with blanket or sheet as if you were about to wrap him totally with it; during this attempt to distract, each staff member should take an arm or leg, raise pt. off his feet & place him face down on floor so that he loses his base of support for physically assaultive behavior; use good body mechanics and be aware of pt's. body alignment to prevent injuries to staff & pt.;
- transport pt. to his room (each limb still carried by a staff member, with the legs carried from above the pt's. knees); if necessary for control, carry face down; protect head; if necessary, one staff member can carry both legs;
- follow facility procedure for application of restraints; care should be taken to ensure that the restraints do not impair circulation or cause pressure to underlying nerves; A PT. IN RESTRAINTS SHOULD NEVER BE LEFT ALONE; stay with pt. & encourage to express thoughts & feelings about the incident; explore the situation which caused the pt. to experience increased anxiety & loss of control;
- remove all items from the pt's. clothing, especially potentially dangerous, sharp items & matches;
- obtain physician's order for restraints prior to or immediately after emergency situation; if physician orders a parenteral medication, it may be given to pt. either at site of loss of control or after transporting pt. to room;
- take BP & pulse Q 30 min. & check extremities for signs of lack of circulation or pressure; offer snacks & fluids; give mouth care PRN;
- remove restraints as soon as possible when acute agitation subsides;
- allow other pts. who may have observed restraining & transporting to ventilate their feelings & concerns about pt. or their own

The Patient who is Violent

3) Impulse Control

potential loss of control.

Patient will demonstrate increased ability to control aggressive impulses:
- see NCP Guide #3:35, "Depression," Sections (1) Sadness, Grief, Guilt, Anger, and (2) Self-defeating/Destructive Impulses;
- explore violent episode or loss of control with pt.; identify why this act was done at this time; did this act have a "payoff" of decreased anxiety or relief of frustration?;
- help pt. learn to identify the precipitating factors that led to his anxiety & impulsive behaviors;
- assess pt's. knowledge of own symptoms of increasing anxiety; health teach as needed; explore alternative, appropriate ways to deal with anxiety;
- explore pt's. attitudes about expressing resentment, anger, frustration & other intense emotions; health teach appropriate expressions of resentment, anger, frustration & assertive behavior; use role playing & practicing assertive techniques in group & individual settings;
- validate pt's. appropriate responses to frustration, resentment, anger & anxiety;
- explore alternatives to over-control & withdrawal using role playing & practicing assertive techniques in group & individual settings;
- make contract with pt. that he will contact staff member when he feels symptoms of increasing anxiety & fears loss of control; plan with pt. for alternative behaviors to control aggressive impulses & express feelings in effective, non-violent way;
- work with family/significant other (SO) so they may understand pt. & work with him to develop & support new coping.

Discharge Planning and Teaching Objectives/Outcomes:
1) (Patient and/or family/significant other) Can verbalize chain of events and feelings that have usually preceded a violent episode.
2) Has developed at least one new alternative for dealing with aggressive impulses.
3) Is able to express feelings in an appropriate way that is not harmful to self, others or environment.

Recommended References
"Assault: Patterns of Emergency Room Visits," by A. Burgess and P. Johansen, Journal of Psychiatric Nursing & Mental Health Service, November 1976: 32-35.
"Control of Violence in Mental Health Settings," by P. Penningroth, American Journal of Nursing, April 1976: 606-609.
"He Acted Up but He Was Only Acting Out," RN, May 1977: 40-81.

"Nursing Aides and Patient Violence," by P. Lovy and P. Hartocollis, American Journal of Psychiatry, April 1976: 429-431.
"The Patient Manifesting Aggression," NCP Guide, #1:20, Nurseco, 1974.
"The Patient Manifesting Anger," NCP Guide, #1:21, Nurseco, 1974.
"Scapegoating," by L. Stafford, American Journal of Nursing, March 1977: 406-409.
"Scapegoating Among Professionals," by N. Wachter-Shikora, American Journal of Nursing, March 1977: 408-409.
"When a Patient Becomes Violent," by R. Anders, American Journal of Nursing, July 1977: 1144-1148.
"When It Comes to Difficult Patients," by P. Sharer, Nursing '77, September 7:36-37.

© Margo Creighton Neal, 1978

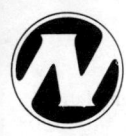

The Child: Battered Child Syndrome

Definition: "Battered Child Syndrome" is the term used by hospitals to identify the victim of child abuse. Child abuse is non-accidental physical injury or attack inflicted upon children by their caretakers. It is damage (neglect, psychological battering or sexual molestation) to the child for which there is no reasonable explanation.

LONG TERM GOAL: The child will experience healing, protection and relief from pain, injury, fear and neglect. The parents (or caretakers) will experience helpful support in adapting methods that limit the potential for abusing their child. The parents will implement new coping mechanisms, will seek appropriate help and will not abuse the child.

General Considerations:
- Common manifestations: a pre-school child or infant in poor general health with a history of previous injuries; includes bruises, welts, abrasions, contusions, lacerations and burns; falls with head injuries are common.
- Causes: child abuse is an adult illness of epidemic proportions with many dimensions: psycho-pathological, behavioral, environmental, social and cultural factors. Ninety per cent of abusers have a history of themselves being abused by parents. Triggering behaviors include: drug and alcohol intoxication, quarreling between adults/caretakers, uncontrolled sibling rivalry or perceived atypical childish behavior, stressful life situations or crises (large or small) with inadequate coping mechanisms.
- Suggested nursing responsibilities include:

  (1) Become informed; read recommended references here; attend seminars on subject; write for further information to:

  National Committee for Prevention of Child Abuse
  111 East Wacker Drive, Suite 510
  Chicago, IL 60601

  The Child Abuse League of America
  67 Irving Place
  New York, NY 10003

  The Children's Division of the American
      Humane Association
  P.O. Box 1226
  Denver, CO 80201

  National Center for the Prevention and Treatment
      of Child Abuse and Neglect
  Dept. of Pediatrics, University of Colorado Medical Center
  1205 Oneida Street, Denver, CO 80220

  (2) Become concerned over this growing problem and become involved; learn what local services exist; compile a resource file for use by other

professionals as well as yourself; consider joining or forming a group of:
- VICA—"Volunteers in Child Abuse," a project involving trained volunteers with parents who need support, friendship and role models to help their parenting skills.
- "For Kid's Sake," an organization that helps detect and prevent child abuse.
- CALL—"Child Abuse Listening Line" or "Parents Anonymous Hot Line"—Be a telephone volunteer.
- "P.A. Buddies": Work with troubled parents on a one-to-one basis.
- "P.A. Sponsors", gives low key guidance and support to PA groups.

(3) Report cases of suspected child abuse; know whether your state has permissive or mandatory legislation on reporting; persons who report in good faith are granted immunity from criminal and civil court action, even if the report proves erroneous; copping out behind a "failure to thrive" or "accidental injury" diagnosis hurts not only the child but also the parents who need help; protecting children and helping parents is the fundamental responsibility of maternal-child health and public health nurses.

(4) Work to develop within your health agency a concerted effort with policy guidelines on child abuse prevention and treatment which will plug into your community services, avoiding duplication and wasted resources.

Specific Considerations, Potential Patient Outcomes and Nursing Actions:

1) Observation — The patient will be observed for findings leading to a diagnosis of possible child abuse:
- note & chart unusual findings upon admission (scars, bruises, unexplained marks);
- observe & describe suspicious behavioral characteristics (passive response to pain, fearful & withdrawn, flinching & ducking when anyone reaches out to touch, violent agressiveness to dolls & play objects);
- observe, assess & record social environment of family (parents' potential for abuse & child's risk: see recommended references for screening suggestions).

2) Protection from Injury — The child will have maximum healing, recovery and protection from further injury:
- monitor visitors discreetly; friendly visits with caretakers can provide acceptance & diffuse hostility;
- follow nursing care plan for specific type of injury (head injury, fracture, burn, etc.);
- make referral to hospital social service dept. or your local Dept. of Social Service, community mental health center or child abuse prevention center.

3) Psychosocial Adjustment — The child will experience relief from pain, fear and emotional side effects of trauma:
- encourage child to talk about how s/he feels; be a warm, quiet listener, avoiding judgmental comment;
- provide drawing materials, as children often depict their feelings in this way; gently ask about meanings of drawings; do not probe;

The Child: Battered Child Syndrome

- provide other play materials and objects for expressing feelings (puppets, doll houses, etc.); refer to NCPG #3:30, "Play Therapy;"
- make a referral to mental health liaison nurse or psychiatrist, if advisable;
- provide for the child's physical comfort with analgesics PRN, with attention to physical needs;
- give comfort by holding, rocking, stroking gently, hugging; note child's reactions/tolerance.

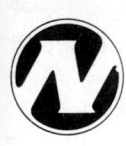

4) Parent-Nurse Relationship

The parents relate to at least one nurse with trust, acceptance of offer to listen and to help and with open discussion of problems and needs:
- be aware of your own non-verbal messages & feelings; communicate those which are positive & supporting; maintain composure & compassion, refraining from even implied criticism or rejection;
- consider asking a mental health worker, psychiatric nurse (who has experience with abused children) to assist you in working through your feelings & planning care for this pt./family;
- be honest with yourself & if you can't handle it, admit it & ask to be relieved of this assignment;
- consider asking parent(s) to keep a daily diary of their feelings & situations in which they feel stress; ask them to identify the triggers that set off a chain of events; tell them many other parents have the same feelings; use the diary as a method to talk through feelings & develop new coping strategies, & lay plans to participate in family therapy;
- let the parent(s) know that you really care about them as persons with feelings that you respect.

5) Parent-Child Relationship

The parent(s) will develop an improved relationship with their child; the parent(s) will express satisfaction with efforts to understand and enjoy their child:
- assist parents to enjoy their child; point out attributes & features of the child that are lovable; introduce the parent(s) to the pleasures of reading to the child, being careful to select materials that will be of interest to the parent(s) as well as to the child; consult librarian for assistance in the selection of age-appropriate materials;
- ask the parent(s) to join you & the child in simple games, doll play, drawing & painting experiences; refer to NCPG #3:30, "Play Therapy;"
- teach parent(s) about normal expectations of growth & development; refer to NCPGs #3:22, 3:23, 3:24, 3:25, "Normal Growth & Development: Newborn, Infant, Toddler/Preschool, School Age Child;"

NCP Guide No. **4:20** 118

- demonstrate how limits can be set & enforced, how discipline can be given with consistency & fairness & without physical force or anger;
- reinforce with praise & encouragement any attempts to nurture, comfort or express affection to the child;
- reassure parent(s) that they too have rights & needs; that there is an organization of parents who can provide assistance in time of crisis & need; assure them of anonymity & privacy; (if this is not available in your community, perhaps you can form a small group of parents who care enough to help & will permit you to give out their phone numbers).

Discharge Planning and Teaching Objectives/Outcomes:

1) The parent(s) knows about, and has written down in more than one place, the Parents Anonymous toll-free 24 hour telephone number (1-800-421-0353 if there is a local chapter of PA, the parent(s) has address and phone number.
2) The child and parent(s) have a referral for family and/or individual therapy.
3) The parent(s) can identify at least two new coping mechanisms that will help reduce or eliminate episodes of child abuse and handle effectively the situations likely to induce it.
4) The child will accept placement in a temporary foster home if conditions at home make this desirable, even necessary for safety. The parent(s) will accept this hopefully temporary measure while they get the help they need.

Recommended References

The Abused Child, by Harold Martin, Editor, Cambridge: Ballinger Publishing Co., 1976.
The Abusing Family by Blair and Rita Justice, Human Sciences Press, New York: 1976.
"Behavioral Approach to the Treatment of Child Abuse," Nursing Times, January 29, 1976.
Child Abuse and Neglect: The Family and the Community, by Ray Helfer and C. Henry Kempe, Cambridge: Ballinger Publishing Co., 1976.
"Child Abuse Can Be Prevented," by Nancy L. McKeel, American Journal of Nursing, September 1978: 1478-1482.
Hear the Children Crying by Dale Evans Rogers, Fleming H. Revell Co., 1978.
"Index of Suspicion: Screening for Child Abusers" by Robert Olson, American Journal of Nursing, January 1976: 108-110.
"Normal Growth & Development: Newborn, Infant, Toddler/Preschool and School Age Child," NCP Guides #3:22, 3:23, 3:24, 3:25, Nurseco, 1977.
"The Nurse Who Came to Play," by Ellie Bushweller, RN, December 1977: 48-49.
"Nursing Responsibility in Child Abuse," Nursing Forum Vol. 15, 1976: 95-112.
"Play Therapy: General Suggestions," NCP Guide #3:30, Nurseco, 1977.
"Prevent Child Abuse," (brochure), National Committee for Prevention of Child Abuse, 111 E. Wacker Drive, Suite 510, Chicago, IL 60601, 1976.
"Recognizing Non-accidental Injury in Children," Nursing Times, December 18, 1975: 2034-2035.
"Rescue Fantasies: Professional Impediments In Working with Abused Families," by Kathleen M. Scharer, American Journal of Nursing, September 1978: 1483-1484.

© Margo Creighton Neal, 1978

NCP Guide No. **4:25** 119

The Child who is <u>Dying/Terminal</u>

LONG TERM GOAL: The child will maintain physiological and emotional functioning with comfort and reduced anxiety during the terminal process. The family will move toward acceptance and resolution of the terminal process, so they can assist in providing comfort and support to the dying child.

General Considerations:
- The age of the child must be considered in relation to his/her level of understanding regarding death and dying.
- Young children may equate death with (1) separation, departure, disappearance; (2) going into a grave, coffin, earth, or water; and (3) sleep.
- Society and cultural values influence both children and adults in their acceptance of death. Understanding of those value systems influence perceptions of and reactions to the knowledge that a child is dying. ("It isn't fair. He never even got to experience the pleasure and pain of growing up.")
- Previous experiences with death such as the death of a pet, another family member, a family friend and/or a peer will influence the child's perception of and reaction to death.
- Children will convey their feelings and level of understanding of their impending death through symbols (drawings that over time are colored darker), through play with toys and other children, and by behaviors such as anger, hostility, withdrawal, apathy, etc.
- The appearance of a lack of understanding on the child's part about what is happening does not mean the child has no anxiety about death and dying.
- Children perceive alterations in staff and family's behavior around them, and may adjust their own reaction to death based on adult behavior.
- <u>Nursing responsibilities</u> include: helping child/family move adaptively through the grieving process; and helping child maintain physiological functioning with comfort for as long as possible.

Specific Considerations, Potential Patient Outcomes and Nursing Actions:

1) Psychosocial Adjustment

The child/family will express feelings, fears, anxieties, guilt they may be experiencing; will verbalize their understanding of the physical health status and the terminal process:
- assess the child's & family's level of understanding & acceptance of the physical health status & tell them that others in same situation experience many kinds of feelings; ask them what it is like for them just now;
- allow & encourage the parents to express their feelings & accept those expressions in a non-judgmental manner;
- permit child to express anger & hostility, but at the same time, do not allow total permissiveness regarding unacceptable behavior as the child may perceive this permissiveness as total hopelessness & abandonment;

- provide age appropriate toys, pens, pencils, etc. that will enable the child to have normalizing experiences & symbolically express his level of understanding regarding death;
- avoid false cheerfulness & evasiveness as this may prevent the child from expressing true feelings;
- at the child's level of understanding, allow discussion of the physical manifestations of the illness, the diagnosis & possible outcomes
- give information to the child and his/her family about changes that are occurring in the body;
- allow family members, friends, peers, to continue interaction with the child; be available to these "significant others" when the child withdraws from their attempts to comfort;
- as much as possible, allow the child to make decisions regarding physical care, setting the time for required procedures to be performed, and participating in daily activities;
- allow the family to assist with the child's care, or if that is not feasible, to assist with the care of other children on the ward (if the child & his family desire & can accept this);
- keep the family informed of the daily medical & nursing regimen so they can be kept abreast of the child's physical & emotional functioning;
- assess the parents' behavior astutely so that when they need support, are unable to care for their child & need to be alone, feelings of guilt will be avoided; seek consultation from a psychiatric/mental health nurse PRN;
- assess the strengths of the parents & utilize those strengths in planning the management of the child;
- provide opportunities for staff discussion of home care so that if this is a viable alternative, home care can be arranged; criteria for such discussion should focus on:
  - child wants to be home, the family wants the child to be home and they feel they are able to care for him or her;
  - cure-oriented treatment has been discontinued;
  - nurse, physician and/or other team members are available for on-call consultation;
- when possible, allow the child & family to leave the hospital for short periods to have dinner, go to a park, attend a movie, visit with other children, etc.

2) Maintenance of Physiological Functioning and Comfort of Child

The child will maintain as much independence as possible in activities of daily living; the child will experience minimum pain and discomfort; the child will ingest adequate food and fluid to meet body needs:
- assess pain & provide medication PRN; use oral medications whenever possible; attempt to reserve heavy doses of narcotics until late in illness;
- encourage the child's participation in ADL as long as the child's energy levels are not depleted;
- use passive & active ROM as tolerated (see NCPG #1:47, "Range of Motion Exercises"); encourage as much ambulation as possible;

NCP Guide No. **4:25** **121**

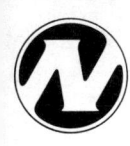

The Child who is <u>Dying/Terminal</u>

- ensure adequate intake of fluid & food; use supplements when necessary & allow child choice of food if possible;
- preserve skin integrity by massage, bathing, use of lotions, sheepskins, water mattress, etc.;
- maintain a pleasing physical environment by allowing adequate ventilation of the room, use of room deodorants when necessary, permitting toys & material objects of importance to the child to be present;
- allow child to wear own clothing when possible.

3) Preparation for Transfer of Child to Home or Non-acute Setting

The child will maintain current level of functioning in new setting:
- assist family members to learn the technical skills necessary to care for the child's physical needs at home:
  - administration of medications
  - positioning, ROM exercises
  - bathing, skin care, etc.
  - use of equipment such as bedpans, bedside commodes, suctioning devices, etc.
- assist the family, and if appropriate, the child, to recognize need for medication & the amount necessary to maintain comfort;
- make home visit to assist family in setting up the home for the child prior to discharge;
- refer to VNA, health department, home health agency, etc. to obtain additional professional assistance if necessary;
- go with family to visit the non-acute setting to which the child may be transferred in advance of the actual transfer;
- assist the family as necessary and as desired, in anticipating funeral arrangements; arrange for social service agencies to be available, & resource persons such as clergy, etc.;
- refer family and parents to self-help groups in their community; keep a list available at your nursing unit for convenient use; the local chapter of the American Cancer Society or Community Mental Health Center also can give names of parent self-help groups.

Discharge Planning and Teaching Objectives/Outcomes:
1) (The Child and/or Family) Can carry out technical skills needed to care for self/child at home.
2) Has expressed some degree of awareness of the terminal process and feelings associated with loss, grief and mourning.
3) Has a referral to a community support group.

Recommended References

"The Child with Leukemia: Parents Help Each Other," by Ida Martinson, <u>American Journal of Nursing</u>, July 1976: 1120-1122.
"<u>The Dying Person and the Family</u>, by Nancy Doyle, Public Affairs Pamphlet #485, New York: Public Affairs Committee, 1974.
"Home Care for the Child," by Ida Martinson et al, <u>American Journal of Nursing</u>, November 1977: 1816-1817.
"I Am a Yellow Ship," by Sheryl Grove, <u>American Journal of Nursing</u>, March 1978: 414.
"Range of Motion Exercises," <u>NCP Guide</u> #1:47, Nurseco, 1974.
"The Dying Child," by Fran C. Northrup, <u>American Journal of Nursing</u>, June 1974: 1066-1068.

NCP Guide No. **4:21 123**

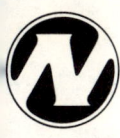

The Child with a <u>Developmental Disability</u>: <u>Mental Retardation</u> (in an <u>Acute</u> Setting)

LONG TERM GOAL: The child will maintain admission level of functioning (or by time of discharge will have returned to admission level) within limits imposed by physical illness.

General Considerations:
- Read NCPGs #4:22, "The Child with MR in a Residential Setting," and #4:38, "The Client with MR in a Residential Setting."
- Children with MR are subject to all the common illnesses and accidents that afflict most normal children. Additionally, many of these children may be subject to more frequent respiratory infections and childhood accidents than other children.
- MR children may convalesce slower than other children, dependent upon their level of functioning, and have similar fears of separation anxiety.
- The physical setting in which the child resides (home, residential, institutional, etc.) may be an important factor influencing understanding of the behavior the child exhibits.
- <u>Nursing responsibilities</u> include astute, sophisticated <u>assessment</u> of child behavior to differentiate between behavior that is due to hospitalization and normal patterns (nursing care time for the non-verbal or limited speech patient may need to be increased in order to assess and anticipate behavioral psychological needs); as well as helping the child/family adjust to the demands and limitations of the acute illness.

Specific Considerations, Potential Patient Outcomes and Nursing Actions:

1) Psychosocial Adjustment

The child/family/care provider will express feelings they may be experiencing; child/family/care provider will verbalize their understanding of the need for hospitalization; the child will adjust to hospital environment and exhibit indications of trust and security:
- assess child/family/care provider's level of understanding & acceptance of health status; health teach PRN;
- encourage & allow time for child/family/care provider to express feelings/understanding in their own unique way;
- accept expressed feelings/understanding in a non-judgmental way in both your words & actions; let them know that others in similar situations experience the same feelings;
- permit verbal expressions of anger at the hospital system & its care of the pt. & if possible, rechannel into discussion allowing expression of real feelings;
- provide sameness & consistency in nursing care as these children frequently respond better to exact schedules & time frames;
- if possible, schedule all care (including medications) so that it will be given by the same nurse;
- try to adjust hospital routine to child's usual one as much as possible;

- follow through on what you tell child, e.g., if you say you will return at a specific time, do so as this helps build trust;
- provide toys, games, etc. that are appropriate to age & level of functioning;
- permit favorite toys, etc. from home or other residence to stay in bed and/or room with child;
- allow interaction from child's peers, family members, or care providers so child maintains his/her significant relationships; most especially ask for their assistance in correctly interpreting pt's. communication & behavior;
- allow the child to participate in decision-making regarding his/her care as much as possible;
- assess strengths of child, family and/or care provider & incorporate into daily nursing care plan;
- refer to NCPG #3:20, "The Child With Separation Anxiety."

2) Maintenance of Physiological Functioning and Comfort of Child

The retarded child will develop and maintain as much independence as possible in activities of daily living; the child will experience minimum pain and discomfort; the child will ingest adequate food and fluid to meet body needs:
- assess child's pre-admission level of functioning; obtain information from child/family/care giver;
- dependent upon level of functioning, accurate assessment of pain & bodily needs is critical to insure adequate food & fluid, as well as minimal pain;
- allow child's participation in ADL as long as undue fatigue is avoided & energy levels are not depleted;
- use passive & active ROM as tolerated; encourage as much ambulation as tolerated; (see NCPG #1:47, "Range of Motion Exercises"
- insure adequate intake of food & fluid; use supplements when necessary & allow choice of food when possible; if child uses special feeding utensils, insure they are present in advance;
- preserve skin integrity by massage, bathing, use of lotions, sheepskins, water mattress, etc.;
- do not wait for call light: plan regular checks so child expects you;
- remain with child until medications are safely swallowed;
- explain & demonstrate use of support systems such as suctioning, gavaging, etc. in advance so when used will not cause fear or be removed by child;
- if child is incontinent, maintain cleanliness of person, bed, etc.;
- measure & record I&O, note BM consistency & frequency, urine specific gravity, to insure dehydration is not occurring;
- observe for restlessness, agitation, etc.; may be indicative of fever, infections, etc.;
- refer to NCPGs for specific disease entity;
teach child/family/care giver any skills that may need to be employed after discharge, e.g., dressing changes.

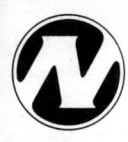

The Child with a <u>Developmental Disability</u>: <u>Mental Retardation</u> (in an <u>Acute</u> Setting)

3) Safety	The child will cooperate with hospital rules and regulations regarding safety at his/her level of understanding; the child will be safeguarded from preventable accident or injury:

- be aware that child may not be able to ask for help & may need to rely on nurse's assessment & judgment on what safety precautions are appropriate;
- check frequently that safety rails remain up; if restraints are necessary, stay with child until relaxed & then make frequent checks; do not underestimate child's strength;
- assist with grooming, bathing as appropriate since bathroom in hospital may not be set up for retarded child;
- plan for other safety & mobility equipment (i.e., wheelchair, walker, other special equipment) in advance so when needed, delay is avoided;
- observe for mouthing of non-food items.

4) Preparation for Transfer of Child to Home or Other Non-Acute Setting	The child will have resumed admission level of functioning (within current imposed limitations of illness) and will be able to maintain it to discharge setting:

- if possible, have staff person visit home or other setting to assess the need for additional equipment or supplies at home, etc., or consult with home health nurse prior to discharge;
- arrange, in advance, for any nursing care needed to assist child after discharge;
- allow child to practice, as appropriate for level of functioning, any aspect of his/her care in advance if necessary to return to home with care still needed (dressing changes, soaks, etc.);
- provide information regarding community agencies that may be helpful to child, family or care provider;
- send home sufficient amount of medications & supplies so the child will not experience any changes in color, styles, etc. of things used in hospital (sameness is important).

NCP Guide No. **4:21** 126

Discharge Planning and Teaching Objectives/Outcomes:
1) (The Child/Family/Care Provider) Can demonstrate technical skills/procedures to be carried out after discharge and has an adequate amount of supplies (dressings, etc.) to do so.
2) Has an appointment for follow-up with doctor/clinic, and a referral to a community support agency (as appropriate).
3) Has a written list of medications, dosage and times to be taken; has medications to last until follow-up visit.

Recommended References
"The Child with a Developmental Disability: Mental Retardation (in a Residential Setting)," NCP Guide, #4:22, Nurseco, 1978.
"The Child with Separation Anxiety," NCP Guide, #3:20, Nurseco, 1977.
"The Client with a Developmental Disability: Mental Retardation (in a Residential Setting)," NCP Guide, #4:38, Nurseco, 1978.
"Maintaining the Hospitalized Child's Home Ties," by Barbara Chadwick et al, American Journal of Nursing, August 1978: 1361-1362.
The Mentally Retarded Child and His Family, by Richard Kock, MD and James Dobson, Ph.D., Brunner/Mazle Publishers, New York: 1976.
Mental Retardation Nursing Approaches to Care, by Judith Curry and Kathryn Peppe, C.V. Mosby Co., St. Louis: 1978.
"Range of Motion Exercises," NCP Guide, #1:47, Nurseco, 1974.

© Margo Creighton Neal, 1978

NCP Guide No. **4:22** 127

The Child with a <u>Developmental Disability</u>: <u>Mental Retardation</u> (in a <u>Residential</u> Setting)

Definition: Mental retardation as defined by the American Association on Mental Deficiency refers to a sub-average general intellectual functioning which originates during the developmental period and is associated with impairment in adaptive behavior.

LONG TERM GOAL: The child will experience as many "normalizing" opportunities as possible in order to develop a lifestyle similar to non-retarded peers. The child will improve physical, social and emotional functioning consistent with mental retardation (MR) level.

General Considerations:

- MR is one of five disabilities commonly referred to as developmental disabilities. The others are: autism, cerebral palsy, neurological handicaps and seizure disorders.
- Read NCPG #4:38, "The (Adult) with MR in a Residential Setting,"
- The term "client" rather than "patient" is the more acceptable word as a child with MR is not viewed as an "ill" child.
- A residential setting commonly refers to a living-out-of-home situation, e.g., nursing facilities, intermediate care facilities, board and care homes, group homes, residential schools, institutional settings, etc.
- Admission to a residential setting should <u>not</u> be considered permanent. Programming, services, etc. should be designed so that the possibility of return to the community is seen as a viable alternative.
- Children placed in residential settings frequently have either profound physically and/or mentally handicapping conditions needing constant supervision. In addition, they may have behavior problems so maladaptive that they impair the child's potential for community and/or home discharge.
- <u>Nursing responsibilities</u> include: working within the interdisciplinary team to accomplish optimal outcomes for these children; and integrating the concept of "normalization" into the assessment, planning, implementation and evaluation of each child's individual program plan.

Specific Considerations, Potential Client Outcomes and Nursing Actions:

1) Psychosocial Adjustment

The child, family, and/or care provider will express verbally or non-verbally an understanding of mental retardation that will facilitate the child being provided "normalizing" experiences:

assess the child's, family's and/or care provider's level of understanding & acceptance of MR; explain & discuss the concept of "normalizing" experiences that promote self sufficiency, adjustment & mental growth, that is, increased contact with non-MR persons, participation in activities normal/usual for the specific age group;

NCP Guide No. **4:22 128**

- allow expressions of anger, guilt, hostility, etc.; accept those expressions in a non-judgmental manner by both words & actions;
- permit child to express feelings, but at the same time do not allow unacceptable behavior, (i.e. physical aggression that will interfere with normalizing experiences);
- provide toys, games, equipment, educational supplies, etc. that will enable the child to increase intellectual, social, motor skills, etc.;
- verbalize & interact with the child in an age-appropriate fashion; though disability may be severe, the use of dignity in interactions is always maintained;
- provide information to child, family, and/or care provider about changes in child's level of functioning; include all in individual program planning;
- allow & encourage whenever possible family members & normal peers & siblings to visit & interact with the child;
- support families through the times when they are separated (physically and/or emotionally) from the child, so that guilt & anger will be reduced;
- if home visits are possible, provide opportunities for families to discuss their feelings about visits; assist them in planning for visits so potential problems can be avoided or reduced;
- allow the child as much independence as possible in activities of daily living; self-worth should be fostered in all activities;
- personal space should be provided so child's personal belongings can be available to him/her; space for decoration should be permitted;
- consistency in care & sameness of routine in events assists the child to orient to time & place; routines are readily learned & provide child with a degree of security & satisfaction;
- when communication is minimal, assist child to develop sign language, etc., so personal needs can be expressed; see recommended references;
- astutely assess for physical and/or behavioral symptoms indicating a possible or potential illness; chart those illnesses that this child is commonly susceptible or prone toward.

2) Activities of Daily Living (ADL); Nutrition and Fluid Balance

The child will perform ADL of (state specific activity as appropriate for child); the child will ingest adequate food and fluid to meet body needs:

- teach & encourage child to perform ADL as long as energy levels are not unsafely depleted;
- refer to NCPG #4:38, "2) Teaching/Learning Needs;"
- ensure adequate food/fluid intake; use supplements PRN; provide food choices when possible; provide correct type feeding utensils to allow child to feed self independently;
- use active & passive ROM PRN & as tolerated; encourage ambulation as much as possible (refer to NCPG #1:47, "Range of Motion Exercises);

The Child with a <u>Developmental Disability</u>: <u>Mental Retardation</u> (in a <u>Residential</u> Setting)

- give meds. on schedule each day so as to maintain consistency & sameness; be alert to untoward side effects which may go unnoticed by this type of client.

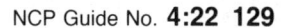

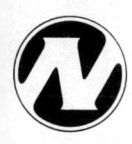

3) Preparation for Transfer (to Home or Other Setting)

The child will maintain current levels of functioning in new settings; the child will participate in the transfer process:
- assist family members or care providers in learning technical skills as well as behavioral techniques that are necessary in caring for the child:
  - positioning, ROM
  - grooming
  - use of equipment (e.g. walkers, special feeding utensils)
  - scheduling—routines—behavioral management techniques;
- assist the child to participate in decision-making prior to transfer;
- visit the new setting with the child & family prior to transfer; orient staff at new setting about child's individual program plan;
- refer child to community organizations which may be involved in the planning & managing of the transfer;
- arrange for the transfer at the best time possible for the child as well as the new agency so minimal disruption of routine activities occurs;
- plan a follow-up visit to child once transfer is completed and a short period (2-4 weeks) of adjustment has been permitted to occur.

Discharge Planning and Teaching Objectives/Outcomes:
1) (The Child/Family/Caregiver) Can carry out the skills necessary to be maintained and/or improved in the new setting.
2) Has visited the new setting and has met and knows the name of at least one member of the nursing staff who will be present on the day of transfer.

Recommended References
<u>The Mentally Retarded Child and His Family</u>, by Koch, Richard, MD and Dobson, James, Ph.D., New York: Brunner-Mazel, 1976.
<u>Mental Retardation Nursing Approaches to Care</u>, by Curry, Judith, RN, MN and Peppe, Kathryn, RN, MS, St. Louis: C. V. Mosby, 1978.
"Range of Motion Exercises," <u>NCP Guide</u>, #1:47, Nurseco, 1974.
<u>Signing Exact English</u>, by National Association of Deaf, 814 Thayer Ave., Silver Spring, MD 20910.

© Margo Creighton Neal, 1978

NCP Guide No. **4:22 130**

NCP Guide No. **4:27** 131

The <u>Child</u> Victim of <u>Rape/Sexual Assault</u> (in the ER)

LONG TERM GOAL: The child will experience protection and relief from pain, injury, fear or physical abuse.

General Considerations:

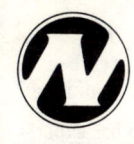

- Read NCPG #4:34, "The Adult Victim of Rape/Sexual Assault (in the ER)," and NCPG #2:35, "Crisis Intervention."
- <u>Sexual assaults</u> on children are usually grouped into <u>two categories</u>: (1) <u>Forced rape</u>, most frequently an isolated, traumatic event, with physical injury, generating fear and pain in the child; child is more upset over the pain and violence than the sexual activity. (2) <u>Accessory-to-sex</u>, usually involving exposure, statutory rape, incest, molestation, but not force; recurring episodes may extend over a period of time.
- <u>Offenders</u> in accessory-to-sex assaults are usually an adult the child knows, most frequently a family member or relative, sometimes a neighbor. The offender usually bribes the child with money, candy, etc.; threats, authority and domination are often used by the offender to generate fear in the child and thus maintain secrecy of the assault(s). Children may not tell anyone of the assault(s) for fear of being punished, blamed or disbelieved, but may develop somatic and behavioral symptoms.
- The <u>major traumatic impact</u> on the child is psychological rather than physical. The child will react to the family/significant other's (SO) reaction more than to the assault itself. The child views the event far differently than an adult and when it is dealt with calmly, will usually leave no long-term psychological scars.
- <u>The ER nurse's responsibilities</u> are: believe what the child says; provide basic crisis intervention techniques to both child and family/SOs; to assist with medical treatment; collect and prepare physical evidence; and refer child, family/SO for follow-up physical and mental health treatment.

Specific Considerations, Potential Patient Outcomes and Nursing Actions:

1) Acute Physical and Emotional Reaction to Rape/Sexual Assault Trauma

The child will receive situational support from ER staff; will be allowed to cope with situation in own way;

- encourage the child to talk about the experience & to ventilate feelings but do not dwell on the sexual aspects; suggest drawing a picture of what happened & to talk about the drawing (often easier for children to do than just talk); do not minimize child's feelings or try to talk them away, but acknowledge them;
- know that these children are often misbelieved; let child know you believe what s/he says, thinks, feels;
- use a calm, soothing approach to child, showing your caring, warmth & interest in her/him as a person;
- reinforce to child that it was not her/his fault, that s/he will not be punished by you, & that s/he is not a bad child;
- explain all procedures to child before they are carried out; medical procedures may be more frightening to the child than the sexual

assault; read NCPG #4:46, "Evidence Collection." ensure that a female (staff, police, family) stays with female child at all times;

2) Reaction of Family/SOs to Child's

Family/SOs will state they feel less anxious and able to cope with situation; will verbalize an understanding of what child has experienced; will provide situational support for child:
- talk to family separately away from child in order to help them sort out feelings of anger, anxiety, fear, etc.; encourage them to ventilate to you rather than the child (child may then feel guilty for upsetting the family);
- know that the family/SOs may vent anger at the offender, or may direct it at the agency/staff, or even the child, especially if the offender is someone they know & like;
- assess their level of coping; do they seem able to cope with situation? are they hysterical? crying? in control? if they are hysterical, be very firm, authoritarian if necessary, to calm them down; provide general support (listening, acknowledging feelings) to enhance their own coping ability;
- help them focus on the needs of the child right now, rather than on the attacker; point out that the child needs loving, stroking, holding, caring, to feel s/he is not "bad," was not at fault;
- reinforce that the responsibility for the assault lies with the offender, not the child; family/SOs may be confused, disbelieving, especially if offender is a family member, friend or neighbor;
- if they talk of the child being "ruined," or "violated," or "she's no longer my little girl," point out that she is indeed still a little girl, the same child who now has a great need for support, love, reassurance & protection;
- tell them the child may or may not want to talk about the assault & that they should let the child set the pace, not forcing him/her or criticizing in any way;
- inform family that the child will be very sensitive to their reactions & will respond to them more than to the assault;
- stress the importance of returning to usual family activities as soon as possible; discuss the benefits of family mental health counseling & provide community referrals as necessary.

Discharge Planning and Teaching Objectives/Outcomes:
1) (Child/Family/SO) Have a referral for follow-up physical and mental health care.
2) Family/SOs state they feel in control of situation and have plans to protect child from further assaults.

Recommended References
"Crisis Intervention," NCP Guide #2:35, Nurseco, 1975.
"Evidence Collection: Rape/Sexual Assault," NCP Guide #4:46, Nurseco, 1978.
"The Sexually Abused Child," by Karen Leaman, RN, MSN, Nursing 77, May 1977: 68-72.
"The Victim of Rape/Sexual Assault (in the ER)," NCP Guide #4:34, Nurseco, 1978.

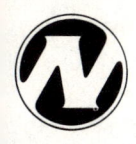

Assessment of <u>Mental Status</u>

Definition: An assessment of observable aspects of the patient/client's psychological functioning.

General Considerations:
- The mental status assessment is a method of organizing clinical observations which provides a baseline for the patient's psychological state; it also provides specific information to assist in establishing diagnoses, planning goals, interventions and subsequent evaluation.
- In the practice of psychiatric nursing, the mental status is an integral part of the initial assessment. The complete psychiatric examination includes a physical and neurological study by the physician, as well as a psychiatric history which includes the statement of the problem, a careful identification of the present episode with the reason why the patient came in at this particular time, a personal history, and a family history.
- The mental status is a useful assessment tool in all areas of nursing practice. Additions to the initial assessment are made by daily observations in inpatient and day treatment facilities, as well as other community settings.
- The nurse may be the first to pick up symptoms of organic brain disease, alcohol or drug use, suicidal ideation, and inappropriate speech activity or behaviors; the patient can then be referred for a thorough medical and psychiatric examination by a physician.
- The mental status examination usually includes areas of (1) <u>appearance and behavior</u>, (2) <u>consciousness</u>, (3) <u>speech activity</u>, (4) <u>thought process, content and perceptions</u>.

Components of assessment	Examples of abnormalities
(1) <u>Appearance & Behavior</u>: observe for:	
- <u>Dress, grooming & personal hygiene</u>; colors, makeup, condition of clothes; skin color & condition.	- Inappropriate to age or place; condition of clothes unusual. Unkempt appearance, unshaven, body odor, pediculosis or other unusual skin condition.
- <u>Posture</u>: describe. Erect, seated, horizontal.	- Stooped, slumped; note open or closed posture.
- <u>Gait</u>: describe.	- Shuffles, limps, fast, slow, akathisia.
- Motor behavior: describe ability to relax and level & pattern of activity; relationship to topics of discussion or activities & people around area.	- Signs of anxiety: moist hands, restlessness or retarded movement, dilated pupils, carotid pulses visibly noticeable or bounding, pacing.

- <u>Affect</u>: facial expression & mobility; describe sad, serious, smiling, immobile, flat (no expression).
- <u>Scars and other marks</u>:

- <u>Prostheses</u>: eyeglasses, contact lenses, cane, dentures, etc.
- Note culture, growth & development, developmental tasks.

(2) <u>Consciousness</u>:
- <u>Determine orientation to time, place & person</u> by asking questions about time of day, date, year, duration of hospitalization. Use direct questioning if appropriate: "Do you get confused at times? For example, what day is it today?"
- <u>Note sensorium</u> of the patient: if patient is aware of his surroundings, his sensorium is said to be clear.

(3) <u>Speech Activity</u>: describe
- <u>Quality</u> (loudness, clarity, pitch, tone, inflection), <u>quantity</u> (pace, volume), <u>organization</u> (coherence, relevance, circumstantiality).

(4) <u>Thought Processes & Content, Perceptions</u>:
- <u>Assess</u> feelings by verbal questioning such as: "How are your spirits? How are you managing? Do you get pretty depressed (discouraged, blue)? How do you feel about that? How low do you feel? How do you feel right now? What do you see for yourself in the future?"

- <u>Observe</u> the way patient <u>describes</u> own history, symptoms, feelings; follow leads provided by patient's own words. Ask appropriate questions such as: "What do you think about at times like these? Sometimes when people get upset, things

NCP Guide No. **4:41 134**

- Grimacing; tremors; Parkinsonism & bizarre movements of head & neck in phenothiazine reactions.
- Birthmarks, operative scars, needle marks, wounds, trauma on wrist, etc.

- Inappropriate behaviors for culture, stage of growth & development.

- Disorientation to time, place or person; stuporous, confused, clouded, unconscious.

- Unaware of surroundings.

- Slow, monotonous; flight of ideas. Incoherent, circumstantial speech with neologisms (self-coined words). Speech is slurred, speech defect.

- Important to assess for depression & suicidal risk. See NCP Guides #3:35, 36, 38, "Patient Experiencing Depression (Psychiatric)," "Patient with Manic-Depressive Psychosis," "Patient who is Suicidal (on a psychiatric unit)."

- Note evasiveness, hostility, anger, elation, tearfulness, distrustfulness, resentment, apathy, lack of openness & approachability.
- Incoherent, disorganized thought; blocking, irrelevance, loose associations, talkative, silent, aphasia.

- Note <u>indications of compulsions</u> (repetitive acts that the patient

Assessment of **Mental Status**

seem unreal. Is this happening now to you?"

- Inquire about <u>feelings of unreality, depersonalization</u> (a sense that one's self is different, changed, unreal, has lost identity), feelings of <u>persecution</u> (a sense that the patient is disliked, persecuted, being plotted against), feelings of <u>influence</u> (a sense that others are controlling or manipulating patient), feelings of <u>reference</u> (a sense that outside events such as TV or radio are related to patient, communicating to patient or about patient).
- <u>Assess for:</u>
  - <u>Memory for recent events</u> by asking about events in recent past; <u>retention & recall</u> are assessed by giving the patient several consecutive numbers and asking him to repeat them. Ask patient to give a chronological account of his life to assess past memory. Ask about birthdays, anniversaries.
  - <u>Attention & concentration</u>: tell patient you want to test his ability to concentrate. Read a series of digits, starting with the shortest set and enunciating each number clearly at a rate of 1 per second; ask patient to repeat them back to you. If the patient makes a mistake, give a second try with different series, such as:

    8, 5, 6, 3; or 3, 5, 6, 8, 2; or 9, 7, 6, 5, 3, 2.

    Ask patient to repeat digits to you backwards. Ask patient to count backwards from 100 by 5's; note effort required

feels driven to do), <u>obsessions</u> (recurrent, uncontrollable thoughts), <u>doubting and indecision</u>, phobias (irrational fears), <u>free-floating anxieties</u> (feelings of dread or impending doom; ill-defined dread).
- Feelings of unreality, depersonalization, persecution, influence, reference, delusions (false fixed belief), illusions (misinterpretation of sensory stimuli), hallucinations (subjective sensory perceptions). Assumes listening or watchful posture; attitude may indicate hallucinations.

- Poor recent memory in organic brain disease or high anxiety state.

- Poor retention & recall.

- Poor performance of digit span is characteristic of organic brain disease; performance is also limited by mental retardation.

- Unable to repeat at least 5 to 8 digits forward or 4 to 6 backwards (the usual number).

and speed & accuracy of the responses.
- **Judgment**: by asking about daily life of patient; note ability to compare thoughts and events, relationships, and draw valid conclusions. Ask: "What should you do if you are stopped for a traffic/speeding ticket?" "What should you do if you miss the bus?"
- **Abstract thinking**, by asking the patient to interpret simple proverbs such as "A rolling stone gathers no moss," or "Don't cross your bridges until you get to them."
- **Insight** as assessment interview progresses; does patient show understanding of his present situation? How does he describe his problems or the cause of his present state?

- Inability to make comparisons of thought and events, understand the relationships, draw valid conclusions.

- Concrete responses may indicate organic brain disorder, schizophrenia, low intelligence.

- Unaware of current problems or present situation. Unaware of mental illness or abnormal behaviors. Unable to link cause-effect. These are associated with neurotic disorders.

Recommended References
"Elements of a Psychological Assessment," by Joyce Cameron and Margo Wilson, American Journal of Nursing, February 1977: 235-239.
A Guide to Physical Examination, by Barbara Bates, MD, Philadelphia: J. B. Lippincott Co., 1974: 306-311.
"The Patient Experiencing Depression (Psychiatric)," NCP Guide #3:35, Nurseco, 1977.
"The Patient with Manic-Depressive Psychosis," NCP Guide #3:36, Nurseco, 1977.
"The Patient who is Suicidal (on a Psychiatric Unit)," NCP Guide #3:38, Nurseco, 1977.
Psychiatric Nursing in the Hospital & the Community, by Ann Burgess and A. Lazare, Englewood Cliffs, NJ: Prentice-Hall Inc., 1973: 170-171.
Psychosocial Nursing, by F. Carter, New York: MacMillan Publishing Co. Inc., New York: 1976: 149-162.

© Margo Creighton Neal, 1978

Behavior Modification

Definitions:
- **Behavior modification** is a teaching technique for dealing with behavioral problems; the purpose is to assist individuals to modify behavior that stands in the way of health and well-being.
- **Target behaviors** are those observable and measurable behaviors that have been identified as behavior problems.
- **Terminal behaviors** are the desired new behaviors to be learned.
- **Contingency** is a term that refers to the relationship between a behavior and the events that follow the behavior.
- **Positive reinforcement** means a desired response or behavior is followed by a positive or desired consequence; reinforcement works best when applied immediately.
- **Aversive consequences** are undesirable consequences and can be used to decrease occurrence of behavior.
- **Shaping** is the breaking down of desired terminal behaviors into a sequence of steps and rewarding each successive approximation of the steps.
- **Generalization** is the transfer of an already learned response to another situation.
- **Behavioral objectives** describe in a measurable way the behavior that the learner tries to learn; they permit an ongoing evaluation of the treatment goals (see NCPG #1:48, "Steps in Writing a Nursing Care Plan," Step 3). Example: The patient will swim or walk briskly 15 minutes every day.

General Considerations:
- **Behavioral theory** indicates that both positive and negative behaviors are learned and that behavior can be modified. Behavior modification includes principles of teaching and learning. The basic tenet of behavioral theory is: *behavior that is reinforced tends to be repeated*. Reinforcement should be given *each time* the behavior occurs; *after* the behavior is established, intermittent reinforcement (e.g. every 2–3 times) maintains the behavior *better* than reinforcement every time.
- The patient should be involved in setting goals and objectives and agree to cooperate with the plan; if the patient has limited capacity to understand this procedure, discuss the information with him in simple terms which he can understand.
- Involving the patient encourages participation, self-motivation, self-care, and limits threats to personal freedom and infringement on human rights. (See NCPG #1:49, "Teaching Patients.")
- **Nursing responsibilities** include assessing the patient for behavioral problems that interfere with health and well-being, and contracting with patient to set goals and objectives for behavior modification.

— **Behavior modification consists of six steps:**
  Step 1 Define the behavior to be modified.
      1.1 Identify problem behavior which needs intervention; behavior should be observable and measurable. This behavior is called the *target* behavior.
      1.2 Determine how this behavior interferes with care, health, and the patient's well-being. Example: Patient is 50 pounds overweight, has erratic diet habits, and wants to lose weight as part of treatment plan to decrease blood pressure.
  Step 2 Measure the behavior to be modified.
      2.1 Gather baseline data, i.e., how many times does the behavior occur in a specific time period? Example: Instruct patient to keep diet diary and write down everything s/he eats for one week.
      2.2 Observe sequence and pattern of behavior; example: Patient's weight is 190 lbs; daily diet diary indicates no breakfast, a high calorie 10 AM snack, a sandwich and malt for lunch, peanuts and wine at 5 PM, and a large dinner with dessert at 8 PM.
  Step 3 Analyse current contingencies that maintain problem behavior or lack of ability, knowledge, or experience.
      3.1 Assess for events that precede and follow behavior; pay attention to feelings as well as to who, what, when, how, and why.
      3.2 Involve the patient and family in this analysis; encourage the patient to count and keep track of behavior and feelings that accompany it by keeping a journal, diary, or chart.
      3.3 Assess for deficits in behavioral repertoire; these may be skills and abilities which the patient has not learned or is not currently using. Example: Patient eats to give self treat; does not know how to nurture self in other ways. Gets up too late for breakfast and eats lunch out because there is nothing in the house to take for lunch. Eats dinner late to eat with husband. Snacks to cope with anxiety and depression. Willing to work on anxiety and depression by learning new ways to cope.
  Step 4 Construct program to change behavior in desired directions.
      4.1 Set and write out behavioral objectives to modify the target behavior to the desired terminal behavior; include the setting or conditions under which the desired behavior is expected to occur, the specific desired behavior that can be observed and measured, and the criterion for how and when the behavior will be performed.
      4.2 Include the patient in setting goals and planning program; the patient can help select appropriate positive reinforcers and suitable aversive consequences.
      4.3 Nursing behaviors for positive reinforcement should include spending time with patient, verbal praise and encouragement, smiling, showing interest in discussion of specific subjects, providing opportunity for patient to have special experiences or treats.

4.4 Aversive consequences could include discontinuing special experiences or treats, participation in chores that are disliked by patient, or nursing behaviors of disinterest, frowning, turning face away, or spending less time with patient.

4.5 Teach patient that all behavior has consequences and that each individual can choose among many alternative actions and resulting consequences.

4.6 Set a specific time for trial run of program and agree to evaluate effectiveness at that time. Example: Patient will reduce diet intake to ingest 1200 calories a day, which will include 3 meals plus two snacks and a well-balanced diet. Patient will weigh in once a week and will be able to plan and have a non-food treat (flowers, music, new clothes, perfume) each time s/he loses 5 pounds. Patient will swim or walk 15 minutes daily. If no weight lost or if weight gained, patient agrees to clean out garage or wash down walls for neighbor.

Step 5 *Use therapeutic instructions (expectancy).*

5.1 Offer specific plan to practice modified behavior; encourage attitude of positive and matter-of-fact expectance that modified behavior will occur. Example: Plan acceptable diet and snacks with some unusual low-calorie treats; plan shopping to include items for breakfast and lunch.

5.2 Break behavior into small steps in a sequence pattern; plan practice of small steps.

5.3 Include some known desired behaviors that cannot be done simultaneously with target behavior. Example: Play guitar or flute instead of snacking; chew gum while cooking dinner instead of tasting food; folk dance or swim instead of drinking alcohol.

Step 6 *Practice desired behavior, step by step.*

6.1 Begin with known steps and then attempt unknown or new steps; choose simple, unthreatening situations and then gradually include more complex and difficult ones.

6.2 Instruct patient to keep diary or journal of practice, including log of new steps and modified behavior, plus feelings and concerns. Steps might include: Buy low-calorie acceptable food, prepare lunch the night before, get up early to eat breakfast, take guitar/flute lessons, prepare and eat low-calorie, well-balanced meals, keep a journal of all food ingested plus feelings and concerns.

Step 7 *Reinforce small, discrete steps in adaptive direction (shaping).*

7.1 Provide information of behavior change to patient, verbally and with charts.

7.2 Reinforce progress, using plan of positive reinforcement; ensure that each step taken toward the terminal/expected behavior is reinforced.

7.3 Involve family and friends in giving feedback and encouragement for steps in adaptive direction. Appreciation is not only much appreciated at this point, but also helps shape the desired behavior.

7.4 Involve patient in keeping own record or chart of desired terminal behavior, thus increasing awareness of own behavior and allowing for increased intrinsic motivation. Example: Patient can keep own weight chart and could negotiate with husband, friend, or co-worker to give verbal encouragement. Nurse can give praise and encouragement plus listen attentively to concerns, read patient's journal, and discuss patterns.

Step 8 *Generalize terminal behavior to natural environment using natural reinforcers.*

8.1 Assist patient to transfer modified behavior to other similar situations and environments by role playing and using problem-solving method.

8.2 Explore and anticipate with patient the natural positive reinforcement that could be expected or planned for with modified behavior. Example: Anticipate and role play dining out situations in which patient asks for fresh fruit or vegetable substitute for high-calorie item. Anticipate camping trip or vacationing with 1200 calorie diet. Encourage patient to imagine self buying smaller sized vacation clothes and having more energy and lower blood pressure.

Recommended References

"Anorexia Nervosa: Patient Behavioral Approach," By S.B. Steckel. *American Journal of Nursing,* August 1980:1471–1472.

"Behavior Modification with a Mentally Retarded Child," by M.J. Roberts et al. *American Journal of Nursing,* April 1980: 679–680.

"Contracting with Patient—Selected Reinforcers," by S.B. Steckel. *American Journal of Nursing,* September 1980:1596–1599.

"Peer Analysis of Interpersonal Responsiveness and Plan Encouraging Reshaping—Pair/Peer," by M.E. Davidson et al. *Journal of Nursing Education,* February 1980:8–12.

"Promoting Urine Control in Older Adults," by D. Mandelstam et al. *Geriatric Nursing,* November/December 1980:251–257.

"Therapeutic Tasks—Strategies for Change," by C. Goldberg. *Perspectives in Psychiatric Care,* July/August 1980: 156–162.

"Toward Reducing Stress in the Institutionalized Elderly—Therapeutic Tape Recordings," by M.M. Alvermann. *Journal of Gerontological Nursing,* November/December 1979:21–26.

"A Weight Reduction Model for Mildly Retarded Adults Living in Semi-Independent Care Facilities," by A.F. Rotalovi et al. *Journal of Advanced Nursing,* March 1980:179–186.

Crisis Intervention: Adaptation to General Nursing

GOAL: The patient will regain at least his pre-crisis level of functioning; *or* (if the crisis has not yet occurred) the patient will respond adaptively to the loss and maintain emotional equilibrium.

General Considerations:
— **Dynamics of a crisis:**
  - A stress or life change event can cause a real or anticipated *loss* or losses in an individual (Review NCPG #1:31, "Responses to Loss . . .").
  - This loss creates a *hazard* (or hazardous situation) for the patient which *can* develop into a crisis.
  - A *precipitating event* pushes the patient from a hazard into a crisis, and may be major or minor; often it is the "last straw."
  - A *crisis* is the emotional response to a hazard, and occurs when the patient is unable to resolve the loss (or losses) because his usual coping mechanisms aren't working or are unavailable, and the patient is said to be in a state of disequilibrium or instability.
— Nurses in general care units most often see patients in a hazardous situation rather than in a state of crisis.
— **Types** of hazards:
  1) *Situational:* Relates to areas of daily living, e.g. physical illness; change in usual role/job; divorce/separation/retirement.
  2) *Maturational:* relates to a person's developmental tasks, e.g. puberty; adolescence; adulthood; onset of menopause; old age.

Assessment:
— The **Aguilera model** for assessment of a hazard or a crisis is based on 3 balancing factors:
  1) *Realistic perception of what is/has happened:* What does it mean to the patient? Is the perception realistic or not?
  2) *Adequate situational supports:* Does the patient have family, friends, someone s/he can trust? Someone with whom s/he can talk?
  3) *Adequate coping mechanisms:* What does the patient usually do to cope with stress (talk to someone? go to a movie? work? drugs? alcohol?). Almost anything, in moderation, is adaptive; in excess, it is probably maladaptive.
— If 2 of these 3 balancing factors are present, the patient is probably in a hazardous situation (rather than a true crisis), and a crisis *very likely will not occur.*

Intervention:
— Intervention is based on assessment of the balancing factors and is aimed at restoring and strengthening them by:
  — correcting unrealistic perceptions;

- providing adequate situational supports; and
- helping the patient find alternate coping mechanisms.
- **Types of intervention:**
    1) *General support:* consists of listening to the patient, allowing him to talk at length and in detail about what is bothering him; *not* challenging any of his statements; and staying with him. This kind of support is usually begun on initial contact, during assessment and helps you determine the patient's perception of what is happening to him (balancing factor #1). When the patient's behavior indicates that he is beginning to adapt or cope (begins to focus on reality; ask questions), support and reinforce reality, answer questions honestly, share with patient how you see it, and ask him to clarify or validate your perceptions.
    2) *Environmental manipulation:* consists of changing factors in the environment to help lower the acute stress/anxiety; and providing adequate situational supports (balancing factor #2): e.g. flexing visiting hours; moving patient to another room; use of TV, telephone; a warm bath, back rub. Ask the patient what he thinks would help him right now; if at all possible, provide it.
    3) *Generic approach:* based on knowledge of responses to a loss (the Grief and Mourning Process), intervention is geared toward adaptive resolution of the hazard/crisis. This approach can help the patient find new coping mechanisms or ways of restoring old ones that have been temporarily unavailable.
    4) *Individual approach:* based on knowledge and application of intrapsychic and interpersonal processes, intervention is planned around the unique needs of the patient in a specific crisis. This approach is used appropriately by mental health workers only.

Implications for the nurse:
Knowledge of crisis intervention will help reduce a nurse's feelings of helplessness when confronted with a patient in crisis; she will be able to help the patient and or family *maintain* emotional equilibrium (in a hazardous situation) or *regain it* (in a crisis state). How?
- She will know that by providing general and environmental support, she will be reducing the patient's level of anxiety and stress so that he can begin to cope with what is happening to him.
- Assessment of the three balancing factors will tell her where the deficits/gaps are and thus which ones to restore and/or strengthen.
- She will know that the first two types of intervention can be provided by *any* care giver, and that they will be provided frequently, for varying lengths of time, throughout the day or night.
- She will know that a higher level of intervention can be provided by the generic approach for which knowledge of the Grief and Mourning Process is essential.

Evaluation:
— Where a nurse has provided this type of nursing care, is there a way she can *evaluate* and *validate* the interventions prescribed? Yes. How?
— Ask the patient. Ask him, "What kinds of things made you feel better?" "Was there anything else that might have helped?" You may find that some of the most helpful things were simply being with the patient; allowing him to cry, etc.
— For application of this information, see NCPG #2:31, "The Patient Needing Crisis Intervention."

Recommended References
Crisis Intervention by Donna Aguilera and Janice Messick, 2nd Ed. St. Louis: The C.V. Mosby Co.: 1974.
"The Patient Needing Crisis Intervention." NCP Guide #2:31, 2nd Ed., Nurseco, 1980.
"Responses to Loss: the Grief and Mourning Process." NCP Guide #1:31, 2nd Ed., Nurseco, 1980.

© Margo Creighton Neal, 1980

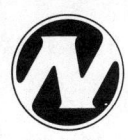

Drugs: Hypnotics and Sedatives

GOALS: To sedate, to induce sleep, to reduce anxiety, to suppress convulsions, to produce partial anesthesia, analgesia, amnesia.

General Considerations:
- Appropriate lower dosages of the drugs below induce relaxation and are called "sedative"; larger doses induce sleep and are called "hypnotic"; and progressively increasing doses bring about anesthesia, coma and death.
- Elderly persons, alcoholics and those with liver disease cannot metabolize safely some sedatives; chloral hydrate, paraldehyde and flurazepam are often recommended for these patients.
- Sleeping pills should be given on an empty stomach as food will delay absorption and desired effect. If medication is repeated the cumulative effect of the second dose will produce excessive CNS depression, prolonged sleep and "hangover" drowsiness.
- When a patient has a PRN order for an hypnotic or sedative, the nurse should assess the patient's real need and behavior basing her decision to medicate on assessment findings. PRN meds. should be given only after this assessment. At the same time, if patients have been taking sedatives at home each night, any attempt to wean them from it will probably be futile. Hospital routine and environments make effective sleep difficult at best so if there is no underlying cause for the patient's insomnia (which can otherwise be dealt with) hypnotics and sedatives are usually justified.
- Growing abuse and misuse of hypnotics and sedatives makes imperative the nurse's major responsibilities of:
    1) teaching patient and families correct use of drugs, dangers of combining medications, side & toxic effects to note and report;
    2) employing a wide variety of techniques to calm and relax a patient, to help him sleep more restfully and to cope with stress more effectively than dependence on drugs; safeguarding drugs to prevent patients from accumulating them;
    3) continuing own pharmacology education in order to know effects of drug interactions and the importance of learning what other medications a patient is taking when hypnotics or sedatives are prescribed; and observing & recording responses to medication, including vital signs, levels of awareness, G.I. symptoms and rashes.

Drug Type & Action	Side Effects	Nursing Implications
1) Barbiturates: CNS depressants: reduce BP, BMR & mental activity; larger doses produce cardiac & respiratory depression	- drowsiness, lethargy, physical & psychological dependence, compulsive use; toxic effects include slurred speech, ataxia & silliness	- teach patient about side effects. - observe & record behavioral responses, ck. vital signs PRN

Phenobarbital (Luminal)
Secobarbital (Seconal)
Amobarbital (Amytal)
Pentobarbital (Nembutal)

- high potential for habituation, addiction & dangerous withdrawal symptoms (delerium tremens & convulsions)
- when given with Dilantin, hydrocortisone, griseofulvin, anticoagulants or butazolidin, barbiturates inhibit their effect or diminish their blood level.
- CNS depression is enhanced when barbiturates are taken <u>with</u>: alcohol, antihistamines, analgesics, tranquilizers, carisoprodol (Rela, Soma)

- know what other meds. pt. is taking & watch for effects when barbiturate is discontinued or lowered in dosage.

- know what other drugs pt. is taking & watch for increased CNS depression; teach pt. dangers of combining these meds. at home.

2) <u>Non-Barbiturates</u>: CNS depressants; little marked effect on cardiac, respiratory or G. I. activity

    Chloral hydrate (Noctec, Somnos, Felsule, Rectule)
    Ethchlorvynol (Placidyl, Serenil)
    Ethinamate (Valmid)
    Glutethimide (Doriden)
    Paraldehyde

    Methaqualone (Quaalude)
    Flurazepam (Dalmane)

- muscle relaxation, low BP, cold extremities

- some fatigue, "hangover" effect
- rare side effects
- some rashes, depression of REM sleep & dreaming
- unpleasant odor and taste, nausea headache, dizziness
- produces peripheral paresthesia ("buzz")
- only minor REM depression

- offer pt. mouthwashes, room deodorant ad lib;
- widely used by drug abusers

Recommended References
<u>Drug Interactions</u>, Revised Ed., Oradell, N.J.: Medical Economic Co., 1975.
"Minor Tranquilizers, Hypnotics and Sedatives," by Arthur J. Morgan, <u>American Journal of Nursing</u>, July, 1973: 1220-1222.
"Rational Use of Hypnotic Drugs" by David J. Greenblatt and Russell R. Miller, <u>Nursing Digest</u>, July-August, 1975: 32-35.
"Sleep, Drugs and Dreams," by Grace Fass, <u>American Journal of Nursing</u>, December, 1971: 2316-2320.
©Margo Creighton Neal, 1977

NCP Guide No. **3:46** 147

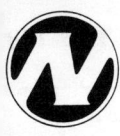

Drugs: <u>Psychotropic</u>

Definition: Psychotropic drugs are those that affect the functioning of the mind.

GOAL: To enhance patient contact with reality and to make patient more accessible to psychotherapy.

General Considerations:

- <u>Drug dosage</u> varies according to individual symptoms, severity of mental disturbance, tolerance levels, general health status, & other drugs being used.
- <u>Nursing Responsibilities</u> include: <u>knowledge</u> of effect, usual dosage, side effects and nursing implications for each prescribed drug; <u>administration</u> of drugs as ordered, questioning and verifying with doctor any dose you question as to safety, dosage; <u>observation</u> to ensure patient has swallowed drug; <u>charting</u> of patient responses and notification of doctor of side effects; and <u>teaching</u> patient and significant other as needed in setting and as preparation for discharge.
- On an <u>in-patient basis</u>, PRN sedation should be used as specifically as possible; an attempt should always be made to find out what prevents the patient from resting or participating in activities and an effort made to remedy the situation. Recognizing anxiety and distress in daytime and coping with the problem before it becomes severe is vital. One or more of the following measures should be taken before giving PRN sedation or tranquilizers: encourage patient to remain awake, out of bed and to exercise in daytime; warm bath; backrub; warm, unstimulating drink; calm and relaxed ward atmosphere; quiet talk or presence of staff member; an extra smoke with supervision; quiet, monotonous occupation before bedtime; eliminate specific discomfort; explore relationship with other patients and staff.
- On an <u>out-patient basis</u>, assess patient's method and regularity of taking medications and attitude about them. Ask specifically: how many? what time of day? does he ever cut down on medication? what does he do if he forgets to take dose? Patient may feel that all medications are habituating or not want to be dependent on drugs; patient deciding to discontinue medication is often the precipitating event to an acute episode.
- <u>Minor tranquilizers</u> are useful in the management of acute anxiety and tension; they relieve anxiety better than barbiturates; are palliative, not curative; See NCPG #3:47, "Drugs: Tranquilizers," for specifics.
- <u>Anti-Parkinsonian drugs</u> are often given with phenothiazines to prevent extrapyramidal symptoms. They inhibit parasympathetic and relax smooth muscle. Examples are: Trihexyphenidyl (Artane), Benztropine (Cogentin), Levodopa (Larodopa, Dopar). Side effects include: toxic symptoms of blurred vision, vertigo, tachycardia, confusion. Benztropine causes side effects similar to those of atropine, and Levodopa may cause nausea, vomiting, hypotension, choreiform movements. The drugs are contraindicated in patients with glaucoma. See NCPG #2:38.

Drug Type, Action & Uses	Side Effects	Nursing Implications
A. Anti-psychotics — the action of this group of drugs is one of lessening the psychotic process & normalizing behavior.	All of the anti-spychotic drugs are considered safe & produce essentially the same side effects. Dangerous side effects do occur but rarely. Side effects may be grouped as: Autonomic- dry mouth, stuffy nose, blurred vision, postural hypotension, constipation;	• Teach patient potential side effects, to be alert to them & to report any occurrence. • Rinse dry mouth with water; avoid candy, gum, etc. as prolonged use may contribute to dental caries.

1) Phenothiazines: most effectively used in treatment of schizophrenia; also may be beneficial in treatment of other functional psychosis, mania, agitated depression & behavioral disorders resulting from organic brain disease. Drug effects are similar in this group; specific drug is chosen to increase or decrease side effects.
 	
    Chlorpromazine (Thorazine)
    Thioridazine (Mellaril)
    Fluphenazine (Prolixin)
    Penphenazine (Trilafon)
    Prochlorperazine (Compazine)
    Trifluoperazine (Stelazine)
	Extrapyramidal symptoms: (1) dystonia- bizarre, involuntary movements of arms, legs, face & neck, often painful; may have difficulty talking & swallowing; onset may be sudden; (2) Parkinson-like syndrome-mask-like facies, tremor, rigidity, shuffling gait. (3) akathisia-restlessness, often difficult to differentiate from psychotic agitation.
	Others: jaundice; agranulo-cytosis; allergic skin reactions; photosensitivity; drowsiness; decreased mental alertness; potentiates alcohol; increases appetite; breast engorgement.
		• If has dizziness or postural hypotension, teach to sit up slowly, pause and make a gradual change to being upright.
		• Reassure that extrapyramidal symptoms are common, temporary and will disappear.
		• Advise pt. to report fevers or sore throats promptly.
		• Avoid sunlight if photosensitivity or skin discoloration present.
		• May drive car, but use extra caution if experiencing side effects.
		• Explain rationale for avoiding alcohol.
		• With all anti-psychotic drugs, symptoms of psychosis often return when pt. stops taking meds.; stress the value of daily meds. as ordered.

2) Butyrophenones:
    Haloperidol (Haldol)
    Fentanyl, Innovar
	Same effect as phenothiazines but less prone to stimulate appetite & less apt to produce orthostatic hypotension.	As above; Haldol particularly good for aged patients.

3) Thioxantheses:
    Chlorprothixene (Taractan)
    Thiothixine (Navane)
	Chemically related to phenothiazines, and have similar effect.	As above

Drugs: Psychotropic

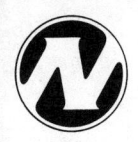

B. **Anti-depressants** - chemical agents that help lift depressions; used in conjunction with psychotherapy.

  1) <u>Monoamine oxidase inhibitors</u> (MAO inhibitors):

  Isocarboxazid (Marplan)
  Tranylcypromine (Parnate)
  Phenelzine sulfate (Nardil)

  2) <u>Tricyclic drugs (non-enzyme inhibitors)</u>: this group of drugs also effective in treating phobic symptoms in pts. with severe anxiety.

  Imipramine (Tofranil)
  Amitriptyline (Elavil)
  Desipramine (Norpramin)
  Perphenazine/antriptyline (Triavil)
  Doxepin (Sinequan) (although not a tricyclic drug per se, effect is similar).

All of this group can produce a toxic psychosis; pt. becomes confused, disoriented and may hallucinate.

A Parnate (or Nardil) & cheese reaction is a hypertensive crisis (severe headache, dizziness, tachycardia, pallor, chills, stiff neck, N&V, fear, restlessness, muscle twitching, chest pain, palpitation) that occurs when pts. take Parnate or Nardil and then eat cheese; can occur when taking other MAO inhibitors as well; also have adverse reactions with other foods and certain drugs, including the tricyclic drugs.

Blurred vision, dry mouth, ataxia, postural hypotension, tachycardia, palpitation, dizziness, fainting, N&V, urinary retention, inability to sleep; profuse sweating, aggravation of glaucoma; stimulates CNS; potentiates alcohol. In large doses, has a sedative action, thus reducing need for sedatives at night.

- Explain to pt. that 3-4 weeks are required for onset of action; teach what side effects to be alert for, and to report any to Dr./clinic.

- Do not give with psychomotor stimulants, ephedrine, epinephrine, or meperidene (Demerol), or tricyclic drugs.

- Advise pt. not to eat cheese, yogurt, wine, beer, yeast products, broad (Fava) beans, chicken liver or pickled herring (the drugs contain tyramine which interacts with some foods). Also wise to avoid large amounts of coffee, tea and chocolate.

- Pt. will usually develop a tolerance to any side effects. If pt. has postural hypotension, instruct to sit up slowly, pause and make a gradual change to being upright. Check urinary output and BM's daily.

- A dose of 50-100 tabs can be lethal; limit amount a pt. has at any one time.

3) <u>CNS Stimulants</u>: give feeling of energy & well-being; used to treat mild depression. Chemical and biological similarity to epehedrine & amphetamine.

    Methylphenidate (Ritalin)
    Dextroamphetamine (Dexedrine)
    Methamphetamine (Methedrine)

4) <u>Lithium carbonate</u> (Lithium): normalizes pathologic mood without sedation or impairment of intellectual functioning. Is used to treat acute mania, and to prevent recurring manic-depressive episodes. Blood levels must be maintained within a narrow range.

Jitteriness, insomnia, decreased appetite; increased susceptibility to accidents, addiction.

Nervousness & insomnia; overcomes drug-induced lethargy caused by tranquilizers.

Minor side effects include coarse tremor, N&V, diarrhea, ataxia, drowsiness, thirst, polyuria; toxic symptoms are: severe tremor, marked drowsiness, confusion, slurred speech, chorea, convulsions.

- Advise pt. of potential side effects and observe for same; teach safety precautions.

- Health teach & observe, reduce dosage with side effects.

- Requires 1-3 wks. for onset of action.
- Reassure pt. that tremor is common, non-hazardous and will disappear. If pt. nauseated, instruct to take pills with meals; tell family to observe for signs of confusion, & report to Dr.
- Coordinate arrangements for monitoring pt's. serum lithium levels (done weekly initially, then usually bi-monthly for maintenance).
- Be especially alert to side effects/toxic symptoms in pts. on diuretics or on a low salt diet, thyroid extract, or those with impaired renal function and CHF.

Recommended References

"Drugs: Hypnotics & Sedatives," NCP Guide #3:45
"Drugs: Parkinson's Disease," NCP Guide #2:38, NURSECO: 1975.
"Drugs: Tranquilizers," NCP Guide #3:46.
"Major or Minor Tranquilizers for Relief of Common Symptoms of Psychoneurosis," by J. Krivada, <u>Journal of Psychiatric Nursing and Mental Health Services</u>, July-August, 1974: 28-33.
"Psychotropic Drugs," by N. Kline and J. Davis, <u>American Journal of Nursing</u>, January, 1973: 54-62.
"Review of the Phenothiazines," by E. Dembicki, <u>Journal of Psychiatric Nursing and Mental Health Services</u>, Part 1, May-June, 1974: 47-48, and Part 2, July-August, 1974: 40-41.

©Margo Creighton Neal, 1977

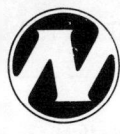

Drugs: Tranquilizers (Minor)

GOAL: To reduce anxiety and to relax muscles.

General Considerations:
- <u>Stress and anxiety</u> are usual concomitants of hospitalization; minor tranquilizers are very useful in alleviating these without a severe sedative effect (as seen in barbiturates).
- <u>Each patient should be evaluated individually</u> re: need for tranquilizers and reassessment should be regularly scheduled at appropriate intervals (2-6 weeks) before continuing medication.
- <u>When a patient has a PRN order for a tranquilizer</u>, the nurse should assess his level of anxiety, basing her decision to medicate on assessment findings. The PRN order should be given only after this assessment. (Many health care workers will give the PRN order without assessment; while this may be expedient for the care giver, it may be less than helpful for the patient.) Tranquilizers do not answer questions which need to be asked by patients about their illness and treatment; drugs do not take the place of sensitive, therapeutic communication which allows normal anxiety and concerns to be expressed, understood and resolved.
- <u>An overdose</u> of a minor tranquilizer can put the patient into a mild coma, but is usually not lethal, unless ingested with alcohol, sedatives or certain other drugs which have a potentiating or additive effect.
- <u>Nursing responsibilities</u> include:
    1) <u>exercising judgment and discretion</u> with PRN orders;
    2) <u>knowing</u> the effect, usual dosage, untoward side effects and nursing implications for each prescribed drug;
    3) <u>observing and charting</u> patient's response to the drug and notifying Dr. of side effects or toxic manifestations;
    4) <u>explaining</u> and documenting drug information given patient and family before discharge; and
    5) <u>continuing</u> pharmacology education in order to keep abreast of new developments.
- Refer to NCPG #3:46, "Drugs: Psychotropic" for information on the major tranquilizers (phenothiazines, butyrophenones & thioxantheses) and to #3:45, "Hypnotics & Sedatives."

NCP Guide No. 3:47 152

Drug Type & Action	Side Effects	Nursing Implications

1) <u>Propanediols</u>: skeletal muscle relaxant (antispasmodic), lowers anxiety
 	
    Meprobamate (Equanil, Miltown)
    Tybamate (Solacon, Tybatran)
	drowsiness, lethargy, slurred speech, ataxia, paradoxical excitement, general CNS depression, physical dependence, compulsive use	• Warn pt. that sedation may occur & to avoid driving or operating machinery until effect wears off.
		• Teach pt. dangers of taking alcoholic beverages, barbiturates or analgesics.
		• Teach pt. to watch & compensate for withdrawal symptoms (muscular incoordination, dizziness) following a week or more of high doses (300-600 mg. daily)

2) <u>Benzodiazepines</u>: CNS depressant, sedative, relieve anxiety
 	
    Chlordiazepoxide (Librium)
    Diazepam (Valium)
    Oxazepam (Serax)
	sedation, lowered BP, increased depression	• Warn pt. that sedation may occur & to avoid driving or operating machinery until effect wears off.
		• Teach pt. dangers of taking alcoholic beverages, barbiturates or analgesics.
		• Observe for postural hypotension; if present, teach pt. to sit or stand slowly & gradually.

3) <u>Diphenylmethane Derivative</u>: mildly sedative, tranquilizer, anti-emetic, antispasmodic Hydroxyzine (Atarax, Vistaril)	drowsiness, dry mouth, involuntary motor activity (tremors), convulsions, potentiates effect of other CNS depressants & meperidine; reports of tissue irritation with injections	• Observe for tremors. • Be alert to pt. taking other CNS depressants. • Teach pt. dangers of taking alcoholic beverages, barbiturates or analgesics. • Use "Z" technique for "IM" injections.

Recommended References
<u>Drug Interactions</u>, Revised Edition, Oradell, N.J.: Medical Economics Co.: 1975.
"Drugs: Hypnotics and Sedatives," NCP Guide #3:45.
"Drugs: Psychotropic," NCP Guide #3:46.
"Minor Tranquilizers, Hypnotics and Sedatives," by Arthur J. Morgan, <u>American Journal of Nursing</u>, July, 1973: 1220-1222.
©Margo Creighton Neal, 1977

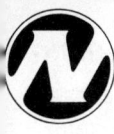

The Effects of Hospitalization, Part A: Tension-Producing Causes

Definition: Hospitalization is the confinement of a person in a setting designed to diagnose, treat or monitor physiological and/or psychological disturbances.

LONG TERM GOAL: The patient will demonstrate ability to participate in his care, make adaptive decisions regarding treatment and care, act interdependently with the health team, and express feelings of sadness over the loss of normal functioning.

General Considerations:
- **Hospitalization** is accepted as a means of treating problems that cannot be handled on an out-patient basis. The level of manifestation of behavioral responses to the dependency caused by hospitalization is a direct result of the intensity of loss of control experienced by the patient.
- **The stress of hospitalization** may intensify symptoms and increase the length of time required for coping.
- **Nursing responsibilities** include assessment of the patient's behaviors, need for situational supports, and the impact of hospitalization on his on-going life style.

Specific Considerations: Common Feelings of Patients that Produce Tension:

1) **A Feeling of Powerlessness**
   - **Definition:** The feeling of the ordinary individual that s/he cannot influence or understand the very events upon which his life and happiness are known to depend. The person feels that s/he has no power to control what is happening.
   - **Some Causes:**
     — Exposure to an artificial, temporary, governing body, such as the hospital staff;
     — threat of force, such as, "If you don't eat, we will start an IV.";
     — threat of punishment for not abiding by the rules, that is, rejection or avoidance by nursing staff, failure or delay in answering of call bells, etc.;
     — fear of the unknown (someone walks into the room; although the patient knows him, s/he doesn't know what is going to happen);
     — imposed restrictions and limitations, e.g. best rest, no BRP, need for help with ADL.

2) **A Feeling of Isolation**
   - **Definition:** The condition or situation of being set apart from others.
   - **Some Causes:**
     — Physical separations from others for a long period of time with no interaction;

— emotional separation from others through use of another language or by treating the patient as if s/he were an object upon which certain tasks are to be performed (e.g. viewing patient as a diagnosis, rather than an individual, equal, client, or health consumer);
— separation from family and friends.

3) A Feeling of Loss
Definition: A state of being deprived of or of being without something one has previously had.
Some Causes:
— Real or anticipated loss of a body part or functioning of a body part;
— real or anticipated loss or change in a person's own view of self (self-image);
— loss of a loved one;
— loss of control over self, others, or the environment.

4) A Feeling of Culture Shock
Definition: The response that occurs whenever an individual is placed in an unfamiliar situation in which his known ways of dealing with the situation are ineffective and in which adaptation clues are absent.
Some Causes:
— Moving a person from a known to an unknown environment;
— exposure to a new language, e.g. hospital jargon, medical terms;
— exposure to a new authority structure;
— enforced dependency and submissiveness.

Discharge Planning and Teaching Objectives/Outcomes
1) (Patient/Family/Significant Other) Can verbally express behavioral manifestations used as a means to cope with hospitalization.
2) Can verbally express those areas of care where s/he wants to be independent and those areas where s/he is willing to be dependent.
Proceed to NCP Guide No. 1:41: Effects of Hospitalization, Part B: Assessment

Recommended References
"Familiarity: Therapeutic? Harmful? When?," by Seymour Shubin. *Nursing '76*, November 1976:18–21.
"From Model Patient to Little Tyrant," by Carol Wiedner. *Nursing '78*, April 1978:36–39.
"How Well Do Patients Understand Hospital Jargon," by Bonnie Casper. *American Journal of Nursing*, December 1977:1932–1934.
"Jack Wanted to Direct His Care His Way," by June Ludwig. *Nursing '75*, August 1975:10.
"Ordeal," by Patricia Chaney, Ed. *Nursing '75*, June 1975:27–40.
June 1975:27–40.
"Responses to Loss: The Grief and Mourning Process," *NCP Guide* #1:31, 2nd Ed., Nurseco, 1980.
"The Patient's Bill of Rights: A Significant Aspect of the Consumer Revolution," by Quinn and Somers. *Nursing Outlook*, April 1974:240.
"Why Did Mr. Howard Stop Singing for Us?" by Nancy L. Bradfield. *Nursing '78*, November 1978:46–48.

© Margo Creighton Neal, 1980

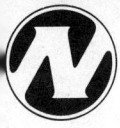

The Effects of Hospitalization, Part B: Assessment

Goal: The patient will use adaptive coping mechanisms that enhance treatment and encourage rapid recovery.

General Considerations:
— **Assessment** is the collection and evaluation of data gathered about the health status of the patient. This data is gathered from a variety of sources including the patient interview. It is utilized to make a nursing diagnosis and plan nursing interventions. (See NCPG #1:46, "Restoring +: An Assessment Tool.")
— **Nursing responsibilities** include the assessment of the patient's **response** to hospitalization, along with physiological and psychosocial data regarding the reason for hospitalization.

Specific Considerations:
1) **Assessment includes** obtaining answers to these questions:
   1.1 What is the patient's usual way of living, loving and coping? (Both past and present ways).
   1.2 What are the patient's past and present experiences that have had a significant influence on him? (e.g. orphan, recent death of loved one).
   1.3 What is the patient's basic personality? (i.e. introverted or extroverted, dependent or independent, pessimistic or optimistic?)
   1.4 What is the patient's knowledge of and beliefs about medical concepts, medicine and medical practice?
   1.5 What are the patient's religious beliefs and how do these influence his responses to illness and medical treatment?
   1.6 What is the reason for the patient's hospitalization?
      a. As stated by the patient?
      b. As related by others: family, doctor, hospital staff?
   1.7 What are the patient's expectations with regard to:
      a. Course of illness or disability?
      b. Outcome of the hospitalization?
      c. Medical treatment s/he will receive?
      d. Care to be provided by the nursing staff?
      e. His family's involvement in his care and treatment, and emotional support?
   1.8 What influence did the patient's method of admission to the hospital have? For example, a) was s/he admitted through the emergency room, admitting office, or the outpatient department? Under own power or brought in by others? b) Did s/he have to wait a long time before getting to his room? c) Was there any contact between the patient and the hospital staff during the waiting period? d) What is the patient's

perception of the kind of contacts he has had during and since admission?

    1.9 What is the patient's initial reaction to the staff on the unit? Is s/he talkative? Withdrawn? Quiet? Asking questions? Hostile? Especially accommodating, cooperative, or submissive?

Taking the data gathered from these questions, plus the data on the Restoring + Assessment form, you are now ready to formulate and write out the Nursing Care Plan (See NCPG #1:48).

2) Writing out the Nursing Care Plan:

    Making a Nursing Diagnosis is the next step. Validate your perceptions with the patient, set goals together. For information on specific behavior problems, refer to section B, "Patient Behaviors," NCPG #s 1:20–33.

Recommended References

"Communication Blocks Revisited," by Sister Mary James Ramaehers. *American Journal of Nursing*, June 1979:1079–1080.
"Elements of a Psychological Assessment," by Joyce Snyder and Margo Wilson. *American Journal of Nursing*, February 1977:235–239.
"Helping Your Patient Sleep: Planning Instead of Pills," by Gina P. Zelechowski. *Nursing '77*, May 1977:62–65.
"Nursing Assessment Form: Restoring +." *NCP Guide* #1:46, 2nd Ed., Nurseco, 1980.
"Patient Behaviors." *NCP Guides* #'s 1:20-33, 2nd Ed., Nurseco, 1980.
"Patient Needs on Admission" by Anne Porter et al. *American Journal of Nursing*, January 1977:112–113.
"Problem Patients Do Not Exist," by Jean Scheideman. *American Journal of Nursing*, June 1979:1082–1083.
"Steps in Writing Nursing Care Plans." *NCP Guide* #1:48, 2nd Ed., Nurseco, 1980.
"Trivia, Illusions, and Quirks. What They Can Tell About Your Patients," by Sandra R. Stafford. *Nursing '75*, September 1975:6–7.
"When Your Feelings Get in the Way," by Lynne B. Jungman. *American Journal of Nursing*, June 1979:1074–1075.

© Margo Creighton Neal, 1980

The Effects of Hospitalization, Part C: Prolonged Confinement

Definition: The confinement of an individual in an institutional setting for a prolonged period of time (two weeks or longer). This prolonged confinement may produce behavioral changes not seen in the early part of the confinement.

LONG TERM GOAL: The patient will be able to verbally express a description of his method of coping with prolonged confinement and self-care activities which make him feel most in control of his life.

General Considerations:
— **Prolonged confinement** results in behavioral changes not seen previously because the patient has not expected to give up control for this length of time. Generally the patient is willing to abide by the "rules of others" when the time frame is short or when s/he expects and prepares for a major change of control. When prolonged confinement occurs in unexpected situations, the patient must deal with additional stress and loss.
— **Nursing responsibilities** include the awareness of possible causes of the behavioral changes which include:
  (1) basic personality needs not being met, e.g.: an independent person is forced to be dependent over a period of time;
  (2) fear of coping again in an environment other than the hospital;
  (3) fear of death;
  (4) sensory disturbances (see NCPG #1:32);
  (5) deprivation of affection;
  (6) sexual abstinence.
— **Nursing assessment** includes awareness of the common behavioral manifestations which are a response to the confinement. These include:
  (1) a talkative patient becomes withdrawn, no longer interacts with staff and/or family;
  (2) a patient who has been actively involved in his care begins to refuse to participate and/or makes excuses consistently for not participating; in his care;
  (3) a patient who has been open with the staff withdraws and becomes passive-aggressive, that is, instead of asking for things or needs openly, as before, the patient begins to intermix complaints and hostility with being nice and saying all is fine;
  (4) a patient becomes confused and disoriented with no apparent physical cause for the change;
  (5) definite personality changes, e.g. an optimist becomes a pessimist; an independent patient becomes overly dependent.

— **Nursing interventions** include an awareness of the patient's need for ongoing control, encouragement and praise of those areas the patient can control, as well as the following approaches:
  (1) converse daily with the patient; incorporate these items into the conversation:
     a. What is the person's level of awareness of changes in himself?
     b. What recent losses or significant changes have occurred?
     c. How does the person see these changes in relation to his usual ways of coping?
     d. What does the patient want the staff to do to assist him to cope with these changes:
        — provide more time for visitors?
        — provide more reading material?
        — read to him?
        — provide weekend furloughs?
        — provide games and someone to play them with him?
        — provide written information about the patient's illness? e.g. booklets, American Cancer Society, etc.
        — provide a roommate who is conducive to sharing time and interest with him?
  (2) Point out the real and identified changes in behavior to the patient; the patient may not realize these changes have occurred. (e.g. "I notice you are angrier lately. Would you like to talk about it, about what may have produced the change?")
  (3) Provide information to the staff on how the patient has changed; encourage staff to be aware of the patient's attitude about how s/he will cope.
  (4) It is important to spend some time each day with the patient; this time should be directed towards activity and/or conversation but it must incorporate a willingness to be involved in the patient's efforts to cope with these changes.
  (5) Fear and feelings associated with a loss or threat of a loss may be playing an important part in the patient's response. An understanding of the concepts of loss and fear is necessary for effective intervention (see NCP Guide No. 1:28, "Fear" and NCP Guide No. 1:31 "Responses to Loss").

Discharge Planning and Teaching Objectives/Outcomes
1) (Patient/Family/Significant Other) Can identify behavioral changes related to prolonged confinement, and ways s/he coped with them.
2) Can utilize situational supports to adapt to continued confinement or readjustment to home environment.

Recommended References
"Instilling Hope," by Barbara J. Limandri and Diana W. Bagle. *American Journal of Nursing*, January 1978:78–79.
"Providing Motivation," by Adaline B. Chamberlin. *American Journal of Nursing*, January 1978:80.
"Survivors of Serious Illness," by Dorothy W. Smith. *American Journal of Nursing*, March 1979:440–443.
"The Seminar on the Chronically Ill," by Rev. David C. Duncombe. *Nursing Digest*, September-October 1975:22–25.

© Margo Creighton Neal, 1980

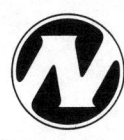

Evidence Collection: Rape/Sexual Assault

LONG TERM GOAL: Evidence of rape/sexual assault will be collected correctly and carefully so that it will be admissible to court.

General Considerations:
- Evidence collection is <u>essential</u> for successful <u>prosecution</u> of rape/sexual assault cases. Because physical evidence is objective and less subject to bias than testimony, it is powerful and persuasive in court.
- Even though a victim may be undecided to prosecute or not, evidence is usually collected since this <u>initial visit</u> is the <u>only</u> time collection may be done.
- <u>Types:</u> 1) <u>Physical</u>, includes the victim's clothes, blood or secretions on skin, scrapings from fingernails, foreign materials (gravel, threads, loose hair) and swabs (vaginal, anal, oral). 2) <u>Medical record</u> documenting findings.
- <u>Evidence collection</u> is done by a doctor and nurse during assessment and physical examination. Familiarize yourself with agency protocol for this procedure and follow it <u>exactly</u>.
- When a <u>nurse</u> receives specimens of physical evidence, s/he should <u>label</u> it immediately and <u>keep</u> all evidence in her/his <u>sight</u> until it is handed over to a law enforcement officer. This "<u>continuity of command</u>" is <u>vitally important</u> in order for the evidence to "hold up" in court. (If the evidence is left alone in a room, handed to another person, left on a desk, etc., a possibility exists for someone to tamper with it and it will be thrown out of court.)
- Be aware that you may be called to court to testify; usually this is just to verify your evidence collection, your charting of the victim's physical and emotional status. If you are asked to testify, call the investigator on the case who can help you prepare as to type of questions asked, etc. Many nurses' associations provide legal assistance as part of membership; if you are a member, contact them at this time.
- <u>Nursing responsibilities</u> include:
    (1) observation, examination and charting of victim's emotional and physical status;
    (2) very careful collection, handling and labeling of evidence, assuring that it stays within her/his possession until handed to law enforcement officer; and
    (3) willingness to appear in court if called upon to do so.

NCP Guide No. **4:46** 160

Specific Considerations, Potential Outcome and Nursing Actions:

1) Collection of Physical Evidence

Evidence will be collected according to agency protocol in a manner that is legally admissible to court:
- explain all procedures carefully to victim before they are carried out (this gives victim a degree of control & a feeling of safety);
- examination & collection should be done carefully & sensitively; forcing the victim in any way may only make her feel she is being raped again;
- refrain from interviewing during the pelvic exam & collection process, as the physical position is reminiscent of the rape/assault & her powerlessness; ensure that she is adequately draped & that a warm speculum is used;
- develop a collection routine that you follow <u>every</u> time, so that you will be able to verify your procedure if called upon to do so in court;
- examination & collection should be done carefully & accurately; label each specimen immediately you receive it; do not rely on your memory to recall where specimen originated, etc.;
- scrape caked blood/secretions into a test tube or sterile container & label as to site; save any foreign materials in a container & label as to site;
- place all clothing in a <u>paper</u> bag; never place in a plastic bag because moisture may accumulate causing a mold to grow on any secretions on the clothing, thus making this evidence unusable; if clothes are damp, air-dry them before bagging;
- keep all evidence in your possession only until you hand over to law enforcement officer;
- after evidence collection is completed, provide victim with an opportunity to wash/cleanse/bathe PRN & change clothes.

2) Recording Details

The patient's chart will reflect an objective, accurate and detailed account of the pertinent data needed:
- describe immediate emotional/physical status of victim <u>upon arrival</u> in your presence;
- ask & record only what you need to know, i.e., information that is relevant to victim's care & legal evidence;
- note accurately statements of victim & witnesses (if any) as memory may later by clouded or blocked;
- be sure to sign all statements made by you; include full names of other medical assistants or law officers present.

Recommended References

"The Sexual Assault Patient," by Gail Abarbanel, in <u>Human Sexuality: A Health Practitioner's Text</u>, Richard Green, ed., Baltimore: The Williams and Williams Co., 1978.

© Margo CREIGHTON Neal, 1978

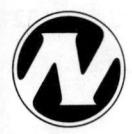

Normal Growth & Development: Toddler/Pre-Schooler

Definition: Toddlerhood is the developmental period in an individual's life cycle that covers the second and third years; pre-school covers from four to six years.

LONG TERM GOAL: The child will develop an autonomous personality and abilities within the framework of the family, and will achieve the highest level of potential growth and development. By the time he enters school for kindergarten, the child will:

1) have had an eye screening test and scored within norms, or have vision corrected;
2) have had a hearing test and scored within norms;
3) have passed a DDST (Denver Dev. Screening Test) for his age at an acceptable level;
4) have received all legally required immunizations (list here for your state);
5) have a record of regular physical examinations and have all current known health problems under medical or nursing supervision;
6) have a dental record of yearly examinations and treatment;
7) be able to demonstrate basic oral hygiene skills and general hygienic practices (handwashing, use of tissues for nasal discharge, covering mouth for coughs and sneezes), and
8) have passed a kindergarten readiness test at an acceptable level or be scheduled to have special educational assistance.

General Considerations:

- Erickson's central problem to be resolved during toddlerhood is autonomy versus shame and doubt, and during the pre-school period it is initiative versus guilt.
- Play in the toddler period is active, informal and spontaneous and frequently centered around motor activity. The principle characteristic of toddler play is that it is done singularly and is called "parallel play," where one child plays alongside another, but not with him. When the toddler learns to give in order to receive, he makes the transition into the pre-school period where play is with other children and is called "cooperative or associative play."
- Safety precautions are imperative; accidents are the leading cause of death, disability and hospitalization during these periods.
- Ritualism is a common behavioral pattern of these two periods where activities of daily living are surrounded with precise activities which add security and stability to a rapidly changing period.

- <u>Learning to separate from parents is an important task</u> of these two periods and is most successful when the child experiences positive periods of short separation and feels trust and security with those who care for him.
- <u>Fantasy and reality</u> become interchangeable for toddlers and pre-schoolers and serve to provide him with a world he can control and understand. Imaginary companions sometimes "people" this world and provide scapegoats and escapes from reality.
- <u>Negativism</u>, or the consistent use of the word "no" for everything, is a product of this period and is the child's way of controlling people and events around him. The toddler especially has a strong desire to act on his own terms and the negative response becomes quite an automatic one.
- Temper tantrums are the young child's way of expressing frustration and releasing anger at people, things and himself in an effort to gain control. An angry, kicking toddler in the midst of a tantrum cannot be effectively dealt with by threats or reasoning for he is oblivious to reality.

<u>Physical Development:</u>
<u>Toddler:</u>
- <u>Weight</u>: 26-28 lbs. at two years; gains 5-6 lbs. over next two years.
- <u>Height</u>: 32-33" at 2 years; grows 4-5" in next 2 years.
- <u>Pulse</u>: 90-120 min.; <u>Respirations</u>: 20-35 min.;
- <u>Teeth</u>: 16 @ 2 yrs., acquiring a full set of 20 temporary teeth by 3 years.
- <u>Body proportions</u> are changing, with abdomen protruding, arms & legs lengthening rapidly and trunk and head growing slowly.

<u>Pre-Schooler:</u>
- <u>Weight</u>: 36 lbs.; gains less than 2.3 kg. (5 lbs.)/yr.; by 5 yrs. is 5 times birth weight or double weight at one yr.
- <u>Height</u>: 40"; grows 2 1/2-3"/yr. by 5 yrs.; is double birth length or 1/2 adult height.
- <u>Pulse</u>: 80-120/min.; <u>Respirations</u>: 20-30/min.; <u>BP</u>: 85-90/60 mm Hg.;
- <u>Teeth</u>: begins to lose temporary teeth (5-6 yrs.)
- <u>Body proportions</u> are changing: loses baby fat & tummy, no waist and legs continue to grow rapidly equaling 44% of total length.

<u>Nursing Implications:</u>

- Parents should be cautioned that appetite and weight gain level off during this period, thus child can eat less and still maintain activity levels, as body requires only 1000-1500 calories/day.

- Due to changing body proportions & rapidly increasing motor skills, falls & stumbling increase during this period & precautions should be taken to prevent injury by picking up loose throw rugs, moving tables with sharp edges, examining toys for safety, etc.

- Due to occasional irregularities in vital signs, heart rate & respirations should be counted for one full minute; blood pressure cuff should be of appropriate size for age.
- Establish good dietary & snacking habits for proper bone development & tooth formation.

NCP Guide No. **3:24 163**

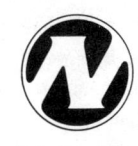

Normal Growth & Development: Toddler/Pre-Schooler

2 years old:
Common Behaviors:
- Gait is steady, walks, runs & jumps with both feet; climbs stairs one at a time with both feet on each step, holding rail. Uses a preferred hand now & can open doors & turn knobs. Can kick a ball without falling, even when running; by 2 1/2, can ride a kiddy car, or tricycle. Coordination improving and by 2 1/2 can throw objects overhead, string large beads and begin to use scissors. Can scribble & copy vertical & horizontal lines. Assists with dressing & undressing self. At 2 1/2, washes & dries hands and is toilet-trained in daytime. Visual acuity 20/70; biocular vision begins to allow fusion of objects & images. Egocentric, he is center of his world. Treats other children as if they were objects. Increasingly able to enjoy story as well as pictures. Has a vocabulary of 300 words which will rapidly increase to 1000 words by end of 3rd year. Uses nouns, verbs & adjectives in various simple combinations & uses plurals; has favorite words & most popular are: "me," "mine," "my," and "no." Self-stimulation frequently observed

Play Preferences:
- Toys: pail & shovel in a sandbox; play doh, clay or mud & water play; climbing apparatus, swings, slides, dolls, stuffed animals, cars, trucks; motion toys like wagon, buggy; construction toys like blocks, beads, puzzles with large pieces.

- Likes manipulative play with sand, clay, play doh & fingerpaints.
- Parallel play predominates.
- Has a short attention span, but enjoys hearing stories & listening to music; likes Dr. Seuss books, ABC rhymes & Sesame Street on TV.

Guidance Suggestions:
- Supervise outdoor play; caution child about traffic safety, fence yard, be alert in driveways. Supervise use of riding toys; keep matches & lighters away from child, watch child around stove & fireplace; use only fireproof clothing. Lock up all medicines, poisons, cleaning agents & store all dangerous tools & garden equipment in a safe place. Teach parent re: poisonous plants. Give poison control center phone number. Use car seat or restraint (seat belts only for children over 44" in height) in autos at all times. Use door knob covers & door locks. Provide constant supervision during water play & tub baths. No popcorn or carrot sticks; watch for choking while eating.
- Child has a need for peer companionship, even if unable to share. Do not expect child to do more than he is able to do.
- Appetite will decrease; do not force-feed; allow child to feed self & have him eat his meals with family. Begin toilet training; be consistent in nomenclature & reinforcements. Use correct terminology for body parts. Begin foundations

as thumb-sucking, ritualism and masturbation.
- Sleep averages 10-14 hrs./day, including an afternoon nap.
- Requires 1000-1500 calories/day; wants to feed self & likes finger foods. Uses a spoon without spilling and can hold a cup or a small glass with one hand.

3 years old:

- Climbs stairs with alternating feet up & down, holding rail; climbs & jumps well; tries to draw a picture, a mass of lines & circles; can hit a peg board with hammer; imitates a 3 block bridge; dresses self with supervision; buttons buttons; can go to bathroom with minimal help.
- Helps to dry dishes, dust, and can clean up a little, tolerates brief separations without undue anxiety. Sentences become more complex, uses language fluently & confidently; frequently repeats words & syllables as a means of learning them. Questions everything with what? why? when? where? & how? Understands simple explanations of cause & effect. Visual acuity 20/40. Sleeps 10-14 hrs./day.
- Needs approx. 1400 calories/day.

4 years old:

- Walks with a free-swinging, adult-like stride; walks backwards & can walk upstairs without grasping rail. Can stand on one foot for about

- <u>Toys</u>: record player & nursery rhymes; housekeeping toys; tricycles, cars, wagons, sandbox, swings, clay, blocks, books, drums, blackboard & chalk; easel with brushes & fingerpainting; puzzles with large pieces; animal books.
- Provide periods for play with other children so can learn to interact with them.
- Provide sufficient space for play.

- <u>Toys</u>: jump ropes, tools like hammers & soft wood & nails; puzzles, paste & paper to cut, sewing cards.

of sex education (see Recommended References).
- Be consistent in discipline & control of temper tantrums; explain to parent the normalcy of ritualism & negativistic behavior.
- Encourage child to brush teeth at least once a day under supervision and at bedtime (done by parents). Take to dentist for first check-up.

- Continue precautions as for two year old, however child does become more cautious about common dangers.
- Give small errands or jobs to do around house, (e.g. emptying wastebaskets, setting table); watch & wait before helping; expand child's world with trips to zoo, market, relatives, restaurants, playgrounds, library, etc.
- Teach him what to do if lost; have child wear an ID bracelet with name, address & phone number.
- Help child express his feelings verbally; accept feelings, even while re-directing behavior.

- Check play area for attractive hazards like old refrigerators, deep holes, construction, trash heaps & deteriorating buildings.

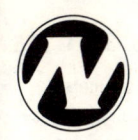

Normal Growth & Development: Toddler/Pre-Schooler

5 seconds. Runs well & hops two or more times; throws ball overhead with control; uses scissors to cut out pictures well; dresses & undresses self with little help: zippers, buttons & large snaps. Can brush teeth & bathe self. Cooperative play now develops; may have an imaginary companion. Is developing a conscience which influences behavior; becomes more self-confident. Brags & shows off, looks for praise, criticizes others and tattles.
- The 4 year old's picture of a man usually will have a head with eyes and two other parts. Has a vocabulary of 1500 words which is increasing by 600 words/year. Talks incessantly; knows name, how old he is & knows the primary colors; scatology (the use of words for their shock effect) appears now. Visual acuity is 20/30 & depth perception develops over next two years; color vision is fully established. Sleeps 11-12 hrs. and the afternoon nap gradually disappears.
- Needs 1500 calories/day.
- Develops romantic fantasies about parent of the opposite sex.

5 years old:
- Can run & play games at the same time; hops & skips well; begins attempts to ride a two-

- Likes back yard gym sets, tires & boxes to climb around.
- Play is more playful-everything is a game; cooperative play dominates during this period; dramatic play (imitations of real life situations) appears and the child wants realistic props; however, one thing can stand for the whole character, i.e. cowboy hat = cowboy.
- Take to children's plays.

- Toys: motion toys like scooter, trike, big wheel, skates, sled, jumprope or hopscotch;

- Monitor activities frequently; know playmates & activities.
- Provide opportunity for group play; invite friends over or use a pre-school. Begin preparation for kindergarten.
- See Dr. every 6-12 months; yearly dental visits; audiometric testing before school starts.

- Teach safety in handling tools, obeying traffic lights, being careful when swimming & around

wheel bike. May be able to print his name. Manipulative skills increase: can use hammer to hit nail on head; uses spoon, fork & knife; may be able to tie shoelaces; handles mechanical toys. Can wash self without wetting clothes. Draws a recognizable man with body, arms, legs, feet & four other parts. Is likely to do what is expected of him; takes some responsibility for actions. Interested in the meaning of relationships like aunt, grandma, uncle, cousin. Has a vocabulary of 2100 words; can count to 20 & knows coinage of penny, nickel, dime. Should be able to sit quietly 10-15 min. to a story. Growth of modesty, increased respect for truth.
- Needs 1600 calories/day.

other toys like plastic toy soldiers, cowboys, animals, dinosaurs, riding toys & building sets.
- Plays house & begins to imitate visible adult roles like fireman, teacher, cowboy; plays cowboys & Indians, war games, and other models he obtains from TV.
- Likes books about dinosaurs, firemen, soldiers, truck drivers, people.
- Seeks out play companions.

flames or heat; never to go with "strangers."
- Prolonged reasoning or arguing usually ineffective. Firm, simple instructions with positive reinforcement should be tried.
- Allow simple choices.
- Encourage imaginative play as this is how the child learns adult rules and roles.
- Begin kindergarten & keep close touch with the teacher to monitor progress. Discuss with parent his & child's attitude toward school and how parent feels he can be helpful in building child's confidence.
- Immunization booster for D.P.T. and T.O.P.V.
- Vision, hearing, kindergarten readiness & general physical condition should be checked before starting school.

Recommended References

Food Before Six and Feeding Little Folks (feeding guides for parents with practical suggestions), National Dairy Council, 111 N. Canal Street, Chicago, IL 60606.

How to Prevent Childhood Poisoning, A New Approach and Accident Handbook, A New Approach to Children's Safety, The Children's Hospital Medical Center, Health Ed. Dept., 300 Longwood Avenue, Boston, MA 02115.

"Sex and the Pre-school Child," by M. Heagarty, G. Glass and H. King, American Journal of Nursing, August, 1974: 1479-1482.

Sex Education and the Very Young Child, Sex Information and Education Council of the U.S., 1855 Broadway, New York, NY 10023.

"When Your Child First Goes Off To School," by Dr. Bertram Brown, National Institute of Mental Health, DHEW Publication No. (ADM) 76-304, 1973.

Why Children Don't Eat and What To Do About It, Your Child's Appetite, Developing Toilet Habits, Your Child and Sleep Problems, and Your Child Goes to the Hospital, Ross Laboratories Creative Services and Information Department, 625 N. Cleveland Avenue, Columbus, OH 43216.

"Your Child's Safety," Health and Welfare Division, Metropolitan Life Insurance Co., One Madison Avenue, New York, NY 10010.

©Margo Creighton Neal, 1977

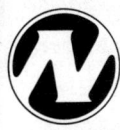

Normal Growth & Development: School Age Child

Definition: The middle years of childhood (school age) span the developmental period in an individual's life cycle from 6 to 11 years.

LONG TERM GOAL: The child will develop his maximum potential within the framework of his family, peers and the school environment; the child will develop a beginning understanding of himself, his relationship to others and the world around him.

General Considerations:
- Erickson's central problem to be resolved during this period is Industry versus Inferiority.
- During this period the child moves out into many different social groups and while the family remains the chief socializing agent, he learns new and important skills and attitudes from his peers: (1) the art of compromise, cooperation and persuasion; (2) fairplay through competition; (3) increased autonomy from the home; (4) reinforcement of appropriate sex-role behaviors; and (5) an ongoing development of his self-concept.
- Play is in groups of the same sexes after 7 or 8 years and "gang" activities predominate in both school and recreational interests: clubs, teams, sports, scouts and neighborhood play groups.
- A form of "cognitive conceit" pervades the children of this period where egocentrism assures them that they are always right and parental fallibility becomes a shocking reality that they are not always right. This conceit can occasionally create in a child an ambivalence about growing up to be an imperfect adult and results in some compulsive, nervous habits like nail-biting, nightmares or phobias.

Physical Development - (6 to 11 years old)
- Weight: from 40 lbs. at 6 years, child gains 5-7 lbs./year (avg.).
- Height: 42" at 6 years. Growth occurs in spurts; overall height averages 3"/year.
- Vital signs: at 6 years are:
  Pulse: 80-100/minute; Respiration: 18-20/minute.
  BP: 95-108/62-67 mm Hg. Temperature: 98.6°F. (37 C.)
  By 10-11 yrs., vital signs approximate adult norms.
- Vision is 20/20 by 7 years, or at its expected adult level.

Nursing Implications
- Urge annual well child visits to promote & maintain health, to teach good health practices; teach children to sit at least 6-8 ft. from TV.
- Refer to growth charts as guidelines, but do not use as rigid criteria.
- Assess nutritional status; study food diary for one week to determine adequacy; ask child to describe eating habits; use opportunity to reinforce basic nutrition ideas.
- Vision should be checked upon entering school and every 2 yrs. thereafter if normal; verify immunization status.

NCP Guide No. **3:25 168**

- Teeth: first permanent molars come in at 6-7 years; loses deciduous teeth in the order they came in, and has 10-11 permanent teeth by 8 years.
- Overall, this period has slower, less dramatic changes in growth with occasional spurts of rapid gains.

- Early development of secondary sex characteristics begins in girls as early as 8 years and in boys as early as 10 years.

- Regular dental hygiene & dental check-ups coupled with balanced nutrition are important aspects of prevention of cavities.

- Children during this period become easily discouraged with slow growth and need to be reassured frequently. Point out positive aspects of development.
- Differences between the sexes are prominent during the middle years in physical and social areas, and these children need support to accept the changes in their bodies; adolescent growth spurt begins by 10-11 years; see references for helping parents increase effectiveness in sex education for child.

6 Year Olds:

Common Behaviors:

- Large muscle ability exceeds fine motor coordination. Very active, impulsive and constantly in motion. Balance & rhythm are good — can run, climb, hop, skip, jump & gallop. Can throw & catch a ball.
- Boisterous, verbally aggressive, assertive, bossy, opinionated, active, outgoing, argumentative, whiny and a know-it-all.
- Dresses self well with little help.
- Knows concepts like right from left, morning & afternoon, and coinage. Can use the telephone. Has a vocabulary of 2500 words. Is learning to read & print.
- Needs 2000 calories/day. Eats three meals plus several snacks.

Leisure/Play Preferences:

- Plays well alone, but enjoys groups of both sexes in small groups. Likes simple games with basic rules. Likes to make things: starts many, but finishes few. Likes imaginary, dramatic play with real costumes. Enjoys running games of hide-and-seek, tag, rollerskating and jump-rope, kickball. Still plays with dolls, airplanes, cars & trucks.

Guidance Suggestions:

- Teach & reinforce traffic safety, provide adult supervision of play.
- Teach child to avoid strangers, never get in an unknown car, never take candy, food or pills from strangers.
- Provide for a balance of rest & activity.
- Teach cold prevention (separate drinking cups) and good health practices, including reinforcement of drug abuses & taking medicines or pills only when prescribed by a physician.
- Give some responsibility for household duties.
- Assure parents that aggressiveness is normal; sidestep power struggles; offer choices.
- Provide wholesome snacks like fruit, raw vegetables, raisins, milk or juices; teach about nutritious foods; have a snack shelf for child in refrigerator.

NCP Guide No. **3:25** 169

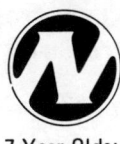

Normal Growth & Development: School Age Child

7 Year Olds:

Common Behaviors:
- Motor control has improved but it is not as important in this period. Capable of fine motor hand movements.
- Is less impulsive & boisterous in his activities; a quiet, reflective period. Begins to deal with the complex organization of concrete concepts: can count by 2's, 5's, and 10's; can add & subtract; can tell time, days, months & seasons and anticipates things like Christmas, birthdays, holidays. Thinks before acting, and thought is more flexible now. Begins to classify and group objects on a general level.
- Cognitive conceit becomes visible. Nervous habits are common. Mutilation, body image & castration fears develop. Wants to be like friends; competition is important. Likes school, considers ideas of teacher important.

Leisure/Play Preferences:
- Begins to prefer to play with own sex. The importance of the peer group becomes central now. Enjoys games which develop physical & mental skill. Wants more realism in his play. Collects things for quantity, not quality: rocks, bottle caps, baseball cards, shells. Enjoys illusion & magic tricks. Likes table & card games: dominoes, checkers. Likes books he can read by himself; also radio, records, TV ("Electric Company"); skateboards and bicycles. Girls this age often ready also for lessons in dancing, piano or gymnastics.

Guidance Suggestions:
- Continue to reinforce safety guides.
- Child will have "quiet" days & periods of shyness that need to be tolerated as part of his growing up. May be subjected to various fears and nightmares; do not permit child to sleep with parent; reassure, comfort but don't oversympathize or give undue attention and importance to these unless they increase in severity & frequency (then see counselor).
- Teach & set examples re: harmful use of drugs, alcohol, smoking.
- Help parents form realistic expectations of child's school achievement, development & behavior. Parents need affirmation that unpredictable & changing child's behavior is normal & expected.

8 Year Olds:

Common Behaviors:
- A return to the active, vigorous & gregarious child with fine motor coor-

Leisure/Play Preferences:
- Enjoys making detailed drawings. Reads comic books, funny papers and books

Guidance Suggestions:
- Safety around autos includes using seat belts, knowing rules of bike safety.

dination acquired. Participates in hiking, ball, follow-the-leader. Movements are more graceful now.
- Becomes a self-assured & pragmatic character on home ground. Eager to absorb the world around him & render opinions on all matters. Curiosity is boundless and he is able to collect and classify objects in a qualitative manner now.
- Increasingly modest about own body.

Strongly prefers the company of own sex, is selective in choice of company and likes group projects, clubs and outings. Uses language as a tool; likes riddles, jokes & word games; now has a sense of humor. Art work begins to show new perception of subjects.
- Needs 2100 calories/day.

on geography & adventure. Likes cards, marbles, checkers, Monopoly. Uses paper mache or clay to create realistic images. Active in all types of sports. Enjoys cooking sets, chemistry & craft sets.

- Needs to be considered important by adults & given small responsibilities.
- Sex conscious: requires simple explanations, honest answers.
- Common problems are: teasing, nail-biting, enuresis, whining, poor manners, swearing; avoid negative reinforcement of these behaviors.
- Encourage to eat, since child is often too busy to bother.

9 Year Olds:

Common Behaviors:
- Cares for own physical needs completely.
- Active, constantly on the go, plays and works hard, often to the point of fatigue. Large group skills & activities predominate, like swimming, dancing & sports. Uses tools fairly well. Uses both hands independently. Rules become a guiding force in all aspects of life. Likes to have secrets, rituals, but less interested in fantasy & myths.
- Strong sex differences in play—much antagonism. Interested in family life, but parents are excluded from a major portion of a child's life. Shows a consuming interest in how things are made; how & what makes weather, seasons, etc.

Leisure/Play Preferences:
- Play is varied, peer activities predominate, like tag, hopscotch, hide-and-seek, statue, dodge-ball, jacks. Books & musical instruments play an important role often now. Watches TV over 20 hours/week. Enjoys handicrafts like sewing, ceramics, models. Board games very popular.

Guidance Suggestions:
- Safety with firearms includes storing them apart from the bullets, handling them carefully, never referring to them as a toy.
- Lying & stealing to gain recognition or attention may become a problem. Harsh & severe punishment should be avoided; try to restrict to room or home, cancel treats, try system of rewards with charts or lists of desired behavior. Understand & accept the child as he is. Know playmates & parents.
- Assess health knowledge & spend time with child discussing health habits. See ref.

NCP Guide No. **3:25** 171

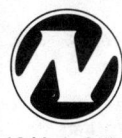

Normal Growth & Development: School Age Child

10 Year Olds:

Common Behaviors:
- Very active with good coordination. Marked differences in motor skills between the sexes appear. Works hard to perfect the skills he does best.
- Is happy, cooperative, casual and relaxed. Is usually courteous and well-mannered with adults. Has a growing capacity for thought and conceptual organization: is able to discuss problems, see other person's point of view, think about social problems & prejudices. This is the peak of the gang age; companionship is more important than play activity. Occasional privacy is important; wants independence. Can understand transformations of state in size, shape, weight and volume. Has the ability to plan ahead.
- Needs 2200 calories/day.

Leisure/Play Preferences:
- Gangs & clubhouse with its secret codes, rules and rituals; experiments in all areas; crafts like weaving, jewelry & leather work; singing in choral groups. Likes mystery stories & TV. Interested in hobbies, collections of stamps, coins, rocks, shells, beer cans, bottle caps, license plates, etc.

Guidance Suggestions:
- Encourage participation in organized clubs & youth groups. Help parents to understand their exclusion from peer activities, but need for supervision from harmful influences (movies & TV, maladjusted companions).
- Continue sex education & preparation for adolescent body changes; see book references. Use "power of suggestion" rather than dictating behavior.

11 Year Olds:

Common Behaviors:
- Inequalities between male & female become more noticeable as girls can no longer compete on equal basis with males in areas of physical strength. Manipulative skills nearly equal to those of adults.
- Is the start of a stormy, active period of

Leisure/Play Preferences:
- Enjoys projects & working with hands in metal craft, ceramics, auto mechanics, bicycle repair, knitting & crocheting. Likes to do jobs & run errands that will earn money, e.g. gardening and babysitting. Very involved in sports, dancing and talking

Guidance Suggestions:
- Set realistic limits that can be tolerated by both sides. Offer support & give democratic guidance as child works through feelings. Needs help channeling energy in the right direction.
- Requires adequate explanations of body changes and special understanding for child that surges

constant activity like finger-tapping & foot-drumming. Is rebellious at routine; moody, resents instruction, has wide mood swings & wants unreasonable independence. on telephone. Likes participation in drama (all aspects including: production, stage manager, make-up, props, publicity, etc. ahead or lags behind. Recognize that they may have a need to rebel and depreciate others.

Peers are still significant; has an intense team loyalty. Participates in community & school affairs. Wants to be trusted and given responsibility; likes to earn money by mowing lawns and babysitting. Boys begin to tease girls to get attention. Hero worship is prevalent. Interested in whys of health measures and understands human reproduction. Can be quite critical of own work.

- Males need 2500 calories/day, female needs 2250 calories/day.

Recommended References
"Annual Well Child Visits," by Sarah B. Pasternack; "The School-Age Child and the School Nurse," by Don Hardin, American Journal of Nursing, August, 1974: 1472-1478.
"Drugs In Our Schools," (and other leaflets or comic books for children), The National Council on Drug Abuse, 8 S. Michigan Avenue, Suiet 310, Chicago, IL 60603.
Fit For Fun and Your Friend The Doctor, by Lisbeth Sanders, American Medical Association, 535 N. Dearborn Street, Chicago, IL 60610, 1969.
Germs Make Me Sick! by Dr. Parnell Donahue and Helen Capellaro, New York: Alfred A. Knopf, 1975.
"Helping Children Grow Up Sexually," Sex Information and Education Council of the U.S. (SIECUS), 1855 Broadway, New York, NY 10023.
How to Parent, by Dr. Fitzhugh Dodson (paperback), New York: Signet, The New American Library, Inc.: 1970.
I Won't! I Won't! (excellent booklet on behavior problems) and Watching Your Child's Health, Health and Welfare Division, Metropolitan Life Insurance Co., One Madison Avenue, New York, NY 10010: 1973. (Also available: catalog, Publications and Films on Health and Safety.)
"Sexual Problems in Children and Adolescents," American Academy of Pediatrics, P. O. Box 1034, Evanston, IL 60204.
The Wonderful Story of How You Were Born, by Sidonie M. Gruenberg, Doubleday & Co., Inc.: 1970.

©Margo Creighton Neal, 1977

NCP Guide No. **3:26** 173

Normal Growth & Development: The Adolescent

Definition: Adolescence spans the developmental period terminating childhood, from 12 through 19 years of age.

LONG TERM GOAL: Through this period of turmoil and rapid change, the individual will achieve social, emotional and physical maturity as a healthy young adult; the adolescent will demonstrate an appreciation of, and security in, his own uniqueness, abilities, limits, values, feelings and responsibility for own behavior.

General Considerations:

- This is a special period of childhood where the individual undergoes numerous physical and emotional changes to develop into the unique individual he has been maturing throughout childhood. Due to the uniqueness of each individual, it becomes difficult to set rigid standards for patterns of development here, yet there is a sequential progression of behaviors during this period and the following material reflects those broad changes in behavior:
- Erickson's central problem to be resolved in adolescence is Identity versus Identity Diffusion, i.e.. . . who I really am, who I want to be, and how am I different from others?
- The critical developmental task of adolescence is to develop a self-concept and identity that is acceptable to oneself and one's significant others. To this end the adolescent "tries on" many different roles in deciding what career, role and personality characteristics are most desirable for him.
- Acceptance is a critical element in the adolescent's pursuit for a self-concept; conformity of dress, eating, activities, appearance and beliefs are all part of his attempts at acceptance among his peers.
- The overriding peer importance of the last period of the middle years of childhood takes on a different character during adolescences as peer groups are no longer isolated exclusively to one sex, but the individual has significant peer relationships in groups of both sexes serving different needs.
- The all-consuming importance for rules of the school age gives way in the adolescent period to a severe criticism of authority and rule and a desire to change the world and make it a better place to live; to this cause the individual joins activist groups and civic change groups to make a contribution and effort at achieving his high goals for mankind.

Physical Development:

- Weight: 95-97 lbs. (avg.), gaining to average adult weight for:
  Females: 119 lbs.   Males: 130-160 lbs.
- Height: 59-61 inches (avg.), growing to average adult height for:
  Females: 63 inches.   Males: 67 inches. (A wide degree of variability

Nursing Implications:

- Intensified weight gain, growth spurts and episodes of fatigue accompany adolescent physiological changes; patient, supportive counseling is needed to bolster self-confidence and encourage sound dietary practices and hygiene.

must be allowed in these figures due to differences between individuals.)
- Pulse: 50-100/minute. Respirations: 15-24/minute.
- BP: 110-118/65-74 mm Hg.
- Teeth: Wisdom teeth usually come in, if at all, by 18-20 years average.
- Development of primary and secondary sex characteristics:
  Female-primary: increase in size of internal and external genitalia; changes in endometrial lining and vaginal secretions; ovulation and menarche (12-13 years, avg. age of onset);
      secondary: increase in breast size, bone growth, BMR; changes in shape of female pelvis; increased fat deposits in breasts, buttocks and thighs; pubic and axillary hair patterns; increasingly smooth and soft skin.
  Male-primary: growth and development of testes, scrotum and penis; production of mature sperm.
      secondary: changes in body hair distribution; increase in size of vocal cords; increased thickness of skin, sebaceous secretions, BMR and bone growth with broadening of shoulders.

- Vitamin/iron supplements are often recommended.
- Caries common during this period; arrange at least twice yearly dental check-ups; screen for orthodontia problems.
- Scoliosis screening should be done and referrals made as needed.
- Questions and curiosity regarding the physical changes in their systems must be answered with honest and direct answers to prevent misconceptions and foster a positive self-image. Listen sympathetically to expression of feelings (worries, fears) re: changes.
- Skin care especially important (mild, unscented soap cleansing with thorough rinsing; use of antibiotic ointments as prescribed for pimples; use of hypoallergenic cosmetics.)

Early Adolescence - (12-15 years old):

Common Behaviors:
- Movement is often awkward and uncoordinated as the adolescent adjusts to physical changes in height and size. Frequently displays poor posture. Physically active, but tires easily.
- Has an increasing interest in the opposite sex. Increased hostility and alienation towards parents or authority figures. Peer group acceptance is all-important; forms strong bonds of friendship with 1-2 close peers.

Leisure/Play Preferences:
- Enjoys activities centered around peer group: social functions, dances, parties, sports, movies, TV, and listening to music; make-up, hair styling, cooking, sewing; mechanical and electronic interests such as working on cars; part-time jobs; talking on the telephone.

Guidance Suggestions:
- The adolescent needs reassurance and help in accepting his changing body; parents need to reinforce positive qualities, seek professional help for problems of skin eruptions, vaginal discharge, dental, drug use, etc. Provide gentle encouragement and guidance regarding dating; avoid strong pressures of either extreme. Set realistic but firm limits that can be mutually agreed up for security reasons; avoid threats; exercise

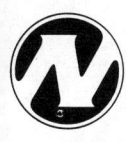

Normal Growth & Development: The Adolescent

- Concerned with morality, ethics, religion and social customs; is in the process of developing own values and standards.
- Wide variations in academic interest and ability exist.
- Females have increased interest in self and appearance. Males are more interested in sports and mechanics than appearance in early adolescence. Prefers easy to obtain "junk foods" such as candy, carbonated drinks, potato chips. Concern over appearance may lead to crash diets or poor eating patterns.
- Females require 2,300 calories/day. Males require 2,700 calories/day.

Late Adolescence - (16-19 years old):

Common Behaviors:

- Will have increased energy as growth spurt tapers. Muscular ability and coordination increase.
- Has achieved a more mature and interdependent relationship with parents. Romantic love affairs develop as a basis for mature relationships. Has an increased

Leisure/Play Preferences:

- Enjoys working for altruistic causes. Sports activities (as both participant and observer) are well-attended. Likes beach and recreational activities like surfing, skiing, sailing, tennis, volleyball and hiking. Reading, TV, music, radio and telephone are all still important.

authority with tact; avoid increasing child's level of guilt and anxiety re: masturbation by letting him know it's "O.K."
- Provide opportunities for child to earn money and have some financial independence. Encourage independence and allow person to be an individual, to feel he has some control over what happens to him; however, be available and allow child to utilize parent, as he needs to do so. Parents need to understand child's conflicts as he attempts to deal with social, moral, political and intellectual issues. Provide honest answers to questions; repeat explanations if needed.
- Provide venereal disease information.

Guidance Suggestions:

- Provide assistance in selection and preparation for a vocation.
- Provide safety education, driver education.
- Provide assistance and counseling in solving problems of late adolescence and early adulthood, e.g., broken relationships, jobs, health and financial.

- ability to balance responsibility with pleasure. Develops an identity for himself and an image of the kind of person he will become. Peer group affiliation is not as rigid.
- Female needs 2,400 calories/day. Male needs 2,000 calories/day.

- Likes challenging games like chess, bridge.

- Parents may need help in adjusting to the loss of their dependent child.

Recommended References

"Adolescents: People, Not Problems," by Ann Lore, <u>American Journal of Nursing</u>, July, 1973: 1232-1234.

<u>Between Parent and Teenager</u>, by Haim G. Ginott, The Macmillan Publishing Co., Inc., New York: 1969.

<u>Food Choices: The Teen-Age Girl</u>, Washington, D.C.: The Nutrition Foundation, Inc. (888-17th St., N.W.).

<u>Nutrition for Athletes</u>, Washington, D.C.: American Association for Health, Physical Education and Recreation, (1201-16th St., N.W.).

<u>Some Questions and Answers About V.D.</u> and <u>What you Should Know About V.D. and Why</u>, New York: The American Social Health Association (1740 Broadway).

"What Adolescents Want to Know," by Sol Gordon, <u>American Journal of Nursing</u>, March 1971: 534-535.

<u>Facts About Adolescence</u>, Rockville, M.D.: U.S. Dept of HEW, Publication No. (ADM) 74-71, 1974.

© Margo Creighton Neal, 1977

NCP Guide No. **2:49**

Problem-Oriented Charting

Definition: A logical, systematic approach to assembling and structuring patient records according to patient problems.

GOAL: The patient's problems will be identified, assessed and corrected through the cooperative planning of medical personnel with the patient and family; a reliable, analytically thorough and effective method of documenting patients' health problems and progress will be utilized; patient care auditing will be facilitated via more reliable documentation.

General Considerations:
— **Idea proposed** by Dr. Lawrence L. Weed in early 1960s; he believed education should enable professional practitioners to be analytically reliable, thorough and efficient rather than to be memory banks. Problem-oriented medical records provide a format consistent with the scientific method of problem-solving.
— **Components** of problem-oriented records include: a data base (medical and nursing history, exam and lab. results); a problem list; initial plans; and progress notes.
— Problem-oriented charting is a natural by-product of the nursing process which incorporates usage of a written nursing care plan. See ANA Standards of Practice and NCPG #1:48, "Steps in Writing a Nursing Care Plan."
— If you are contemplating using this system in your facility, we suggest you thoroughly acquaint yourself with the literature on this subject, attend seminars on Problem-Oriented Charting, talk to others who are using it, and then work with others in your facility to develop policies and procedures needed for smooth implementation and usage.

Specific Considerations, Potential Patient Outcomes, and Nursing Actions:

1) Data Base — A specific, well-defined body of patient information will be provided for the purpose of determining a patient's health problems:
   — obtain a complete nursing history which includes present and past illnesses, health habits & psychosocial data that may affect pt.'s treatment or nursing care; refer to NCPG #4:41, "Assessment of Mental Status," NCPGs #4:47, 48, 49, 50, "Physical Assessment, Parts A, B, C & D," or NCPG #3:19, "The Child: Nursing Assessment Guide";
   — refer to NCPG #1:44, "Suggestions for Interviewing," and NCPG #1:46, "RESTORING +—An Assessment Tool";
   — know that the "data base" corresponds to the first step of the nursing process: *interviewing and gathering information.*

2) Problem List — Patient health problems relevant to nursing intervention will be identified:
   — consider for inclusion: health hazards, allergies, abnormal signs/symptoms, social or behavioral problems, family problems which affect the patient's illness or recovery, and needs for assistance with activities of daily living or health teaching;

- see NCPG #2:46 "Nursing Diagnoses: Tentative List";
- give each problem a date (when identified), a sequential number & a succinct title; compile a list & attach to the front of the chart; have list differentiate between "active/current" problems and "inactive/resolved" problems;
- update & improve definition or statement of problem when more information becomes available;
- when a problem is resolved or redefined, the old problem number is not reused;
- group, if desired, related problems (such as health teaching needs or various aspects of activities of daily living);
- know that the "problem list" corresponds to second step of the nursing process: *identifying the patient's needs/problems/concerns, i.e. the nursing diagnosis.*

3) Initial Plans

A standardized format will be provided that indicates a desired outcome and the methods to be used to achieve this:
- incorporate into the initial plan for each problem, provisions for answering three questions:
  (1) What else do I need to know about this problem? (diagnostic tests, further interviewing & observations to be made)
  (2) What can I do about resolving the problem now? (specific medical and nursing orders, counseling and care)
  (3) What will I tell the patient/family about the plans for solving this problem? (patient/family educational measures)
- the "initial plan" may be written in regular NCP format; see NCPG #1:48; use ink for entries, initial & date them (the nursing care plan of problem oriented chart becomes a permanent record);
- specify clear, measurable & realistic objectives or goals (desired outcomes) for each problem identified;
- state several specific nursing actions/approaches to achieve the desired results or goals; establish priorities of actions, considering therapeutic goals, basic human needs within the context of this unique individual patient, & standards of nursing practice;
- this initial NCP may be written directly on the progress notes or on the Kardex card; if the latter, a notation to this effect must be on the progress notes to ensure a complete record, & the Kardex card must become a part of the chart after discharge;
- know that completion of the "initial plan" corresponds to the third & fourth steps of the nursing process: *specifying goals and objectives & prescribing nursing actions.*

4) Progress Notes

Pertinent changes in the problem's status or increments of progress in the patient's response to the treatment plan will be recorded accurately and clearly:
- progress notes may be charted in one of three forms:

- (1) *Flow sheets* (graphic-type sheets) to record acute or chronic problems which have many components, treatments, nursing actions and/or repetitive observations & measurements, e.g. vital signs, neuro checks; (the type of form most satisfactory is probably one you develop to meet specific needs of the unit);
- (2) standardized *SOAP* format, to be used for writing progress notes on a problem already identified:
  S-ubjective information: what the pt./family *says* about the problem; symptoms, complaints, etc.;
  O-bjective information: *professional observations,* lab & X–ray reports, various measurements, vital signs;
  A-ssessment of Problem: your interpretation, evaluation of the pt.'s response to care, i.e. has the problem changed? how? (increased, decreased, modified by new factors?);
  P-lan for follow-up of Problem: what should be done next?
— a popular suggestion now is to include I-E-R after the S-O-A-P note:
  I-ntervention or
  I-mplementation: measures accomplished for the pt. to alleviate problem;
  E-valuation: how effective was the measure and what was the pt.'s response?
  R-evision: how should the care plan now be changed?
- (3) *Narrative Notes:* written summaries of incidents, accidents, temporary problems, or current pt. situations (return from recovery room, weekend pass from hospital, etc.); title these "miscellaneous" notes: "accident" (or whatever), & chart sequentially on the progress notes, including a date, time & signature;
— when do you chart a progress note?
  (1) on admission (narrative type);
  (2) whenever you wish to record a measurement, etc. (flow sheet);
  (3) whenever there is a change in pt. status or condition (SOAP format);
  (4) *at least* once a week in acute hospitals, and *at least* once a month in extended care facilities (narrative or SOAP type);
  (5) whenever the pt. is transferred to another unit, health facility, or is discharged (narrative type).
— write all progress notes on the same progress sheet in timed sequence; give date, time, problem number & title;
— when problems are resolved, so state under the "P" of SOAP and mark it "resolved" on the problem list with the date & your name;
— if the problem is not resolved, but you are changing some aspect of the nursing approach, so state under "P" of SOAP note & change it on the Kardex care plan with the date & your name/initials;

- know that the assessment/evaluation of the pt.'s problems & revision of the plan as needed correspond to the fifth & sixth steps of the nursing process: *implementing nursing actions and evaluating patient response to care;*
- upon discharge or transfer, all problems, current & resolved, are reviewed & summarized by the physician, nurse & other professionals who have identified problems for that pt.; a separate chart form is usually provided for this purpose, or it may be recorded on the progress notes; if pt. is being transferred to a convalescent hospital, rehabilitation center or nursing home, make sure a copy of the discharge summary is sent; include data which will be most helpful to the health care staff; provide a copy of the instruction sheet(s) given to pt. & family along with a summary of the educational outcomes that were achieved.

Recommended References

"A Visiting Nurse in a Problem-Oriented Group Practice," by Martha Reines. *American Journal of Nursing,* July 1979:1225, 1226.
"Assessment of Mental Status." NCP Guide #4:41, Nurseco, 1978.
"Handbook of Problem Orientation for Nurses." Medical Center Hospital of Vermont, Burlington, VT 05401.
"Let's Set the Record Straight," by Mary Reilly. *Nursing '79,* January 1979:56–61.
"Nursing Diagnoses: Tentative List." NCP Guide #2:47, 2nd Ed., Nurseco, 1980.
"Patient-Oriented Recording—A Better System for Ambulatory Settings," by Betty Ansley. *Nursing '75,* August 1975:52, 53.
"Physical Assessment, Parts A, B, C & D." NCP Guides #4:47, 48, 49, 50, Nurseco, 1978.
"Problem-Oriented Record-Uniting the Team for Total Care," by Alice Robinson. *RN,* June 1975:23–28.
"RESTORING +—An Assessment Tool." NCP Guide #1:46, 2nd Ed., Nurseco, 1980.
Standards for Nursing Practice. Kansas City, MO: American Nurses' Association
"Steps In Writing Nursing Care Plans." NCP Guide #1:48, 2nd Ed., Nurseco, 1980.
"Suggestions for Interviewing." NCP Guide #1:44, 2nd Ed., Nurseco, 1980.
"The Child: Nursing Assessment Guide." NCP Guide #3:19, Nurseco, 1977.

© Margo Creighton Neal, 1980

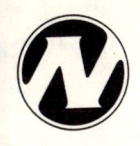

Problem Solving

*"Feed a man a fish and he will eat for a night,
Teach a man how to fish and he will eat for the rest of his life."*
— *Anonymous*

Definition: A systematic method of reasoning or organizing data in order to find useful and effective alternative ways to cope with a situation, need, or concern that constitutes a problem.

LONG TERM GOAL: The patient/client/staff member will learn and demonstrate the steps and methods of problem solving; the patient/client/staff member will demonstrate increased ability to solve problem.

General Considerations:
— Effective problem solving is essential to mental health and is a learned behavior; with practice, the learner can improve problem-solving ability; problem solving can be done alone, with one other, or in a group.
— Behaviors that may indicate a need for problem solving include:

- physical discomfort
- powerlessness
- shame or stigma
- passivity
- incompetence in coping with ADL (activities of daily living)

- conflict
- emotional threat
- hopelessness
- increased stress
- non-assertion
- distorted reality testing

- anxiety
- low self-esteem
- frustration
- guilt
- immaturity
- aggression

— **Components** of problem solving are: awareness of problem area, problem definition, data collection and analysis, formulation of alternative solutions, discussion of possible consequences, selection of best alternative, implementation of trial run, evaluation, and summary.

— **Nursing responsibilities** include a knowledge of problem-solving methods and assessment of patient/client/staff members for unresolved problems that require nursing intervention.

Specific Considerations, Potential Patient Outcomes, and Nursing Actions:

1) Awareness of the Problem Area

    The patient/client/staff member will see, hear, feel, or experience awareness of specific situation or problem area:
    — focus on situation, need or concern; ask person to recall & describe details, including feelings & issues, what was seen & heard, who was involved, when & how event occurred;
    — know that awareness is the first step of change; listen & explore without giving advice or jumping to conclusions.

2) Problem Definition

    The problem(s) will be identified and defined; goals/objectives/expected outcomes will be specified:
    — define needs & goals/objectives/expected outcomes; set priorities in terms of most pressing problems;
    — identify issues & different aspects involved; separate complex problems into subgroups;
    — determine what creates the problem by asking: "Why is it a problem? Who is affected by this? Who else is involved? Who else could be involved in problem solving? Why am I motivated to change the situation?"
    — identify who, what, when, where & which; ask open-ended questions, i.e., "How do you manage _____?" "What is it about this situation that concerns you?"

3) Data Collection and Analysis

    Data will be collected, organized, and analyzed in an appropriate way:
    — decide on a method to collect data which is relevant to the situation (e.g., literature search; create data collection tool to be used to interview in person, by mail, or by telephone survey); problem solving group may be created to bring together individuals with similar problem to share information & offer group support, encouragement;
    — organize & classify data, using outline or numbering method; large file cards or computer system may be helpful;
    — validate findings with other persons; clarify issues; identify gaps or discrepancies in information;
    — analyze data by discussion, comparing & contrasting issues & information;
    — interpretation of data involves making a relationship between facts, using the process of induction or deduction to form a conclusion; identify causes of problem & influencing factors.

4) Alternative Solutions

    Alternative solutions will be formulated and discussed with consideration of possible consequences:
    — formulate tentative alternative solutions, using data analysis & conclusions; consider all possible courses of action; list each as a possible solution;
    — discuss each alternative & identify its possible consequences, including pros & cons, strengths & weaknesses; role play alternatives, paying attention to feelings & physiologic responses;
    — be aware of person's attitudes, values, & feelings which influence determination of pros & cons;

	— assess for lack of knowledge or experience to initiate alternative; health teach as needed in assertiveness, communication skills, interpersonal relationship skills.
5) Trial Run and Evaluation	An alternative solution will be chosen and a trial run will be implemented and evaluated: — choose one possible solution that seems most appropriate; plan and initiate trial run; complex plans should be broken down into small steps; — identify specific actions to be taken; assess knowledge & skills needed to obtain PRN; estimate time needed & anticipate factors that may facilitate or hinder the action; — know that trial runs usually have to be modified or revised; continue collecting data to revise or modify as needed; — be flexible & open-minded; if the alternative is not satisfactory, try another one. *There are always other alternatives!* You may find that you need to start back at the first or second step with awareness & redefinition of the problem; — evaluate effectiveness of alternative solution in relation to the previously set goals and objectives.
6) Summary	The problem-solving method will be summarized, including problem-solving process and content; anticipatory guidance will be offered to cope with next problem: — summarize the problem-solving process, using the problem-solving components & the specific content; this may be done verbally or with charts, graphs, audio visuals, or written reports may be created to share the conclusion or results with others; — identify future situations which may be potential problem areas & use anticipatory guidance to apply conclusions, alternative solutions, or problem-solving methods to these situations; give positive reinforcement for ability to apply new knowledge to potential problem situations; — recognize & give verbal & non-verbal positive reinforcement for willingness to learn & use problem-solving methods & for demonstrations of increased ability to problem solve.

Recommended References

"Behavior Modification." *NCP Guide #5:37*, Nurseco, 1981.
"The Liaison Nurse: Centralizing Problem-Solving," by B.M. LeClear. *Supervisor Nurse,* March 1980:42–43.
"Meeting the Challenge of Fistulas and Draining Wounds," by Sr. V. Taylor. *Nursing '80,* June 1980:45–51.
"Nursing Decisions . . . Stroke!" by M.J. Stillman. *RN,* November 1979:49–56.
"The Patient Experiencing Guilt." *NCP Guide #5:31,* Nurseco, 1981.
"The Patient Experiencing a Threat to Self-Esteem." *NCP Guide #5:32,* Nurseco, 1981.

"The Patient Experiencing Powerlessness." *NCP Guide #5:34,* Nurseco, 1981.
"The Patient Experiencing Shame/Embarrassment." *NCP Guide #5:35,* Nurseco, 1981.
"Problem-Oriented Charting." *NCP Guide #2:49,* 2nd Ed., Nurseco, 1980.
"Suggestions for Interviewing." *NCP Guide #1:44,* 2nd Ed., Nurseco, 1980.

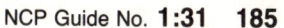

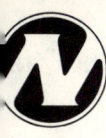

Responses to Loss: The Grief and Mourning Process

Definitions: Loss—removal of something/someone of great value to the person.
Grief—the emotional responses that follow the perception, or anticipation, of a loss.
Mourning—the psychological processes that result following a loss.
Grief and Mourning Process—the process of coping with and adapting to the loss.

LONG TERM GOAL: The patient will be able to cope with the loss by completing each stage of the grief and mourning process.

General Considerations:
— There are **three categories of loss:**
  (1) sexual role identity, e.g. loss of family role, career role, sexual functioning, control over one's life;
  (2) self-image, e.g. loss of a leg, bowel functioning, self-respect;
  (3) nurturing, e.g. loss of a significant other.
  An actual or anticipated loss in any of these categories will trigger the grief and mourning process.
— The grief and mourning process involves **three stages,** according to Engel (see Recommended References): 1) shock and disbelief, 2) developing awareness of the loss, and 3) restitution.
— Each stage has its own **adaptive and maladaptive responses,** and time frame:
  (1) **Shock and disbelief:** Almost any behavior that helps the patient cope with the loss is *adaptive* for this stage. Common ones are denial, anger, crying, screaming; any kind of destructive behavior is *maladaptive*. This stage usually lasts *1-7 days;* after this time, the former adaptive behaviors may be considered maladaptive because the patient has not moved into the next stage.
  (2) **Developing awareness of the loss:** *Adaptive* behaviors are those which indicate beginning acknowledgement of the loss, e.g. "Maybe I will look OK with a prosthesis." "Do you think I'll be able to work with this?" Often the patient's behavior will swing "up" (as above) to "down" ("No, I'll never be able to cope with this."). Patients frequently blame themselves in this stage ("If only I had done . . ."). Any of the adaptive behaviors of stage one, as long as they are *interspersed* with this new behavior, are adaptive for this second stage. Destructive behavior is always maladaptive. This stage can last from *several weeks to months*.
  (3) **Restitution:** In this stage, the patient is able to recognize and deal with the loss, can put it aside and go on with the business of living. Typical behaviors include: making plans for the future; recalling comfortably and realistically both pleasures and disappointments associated with the loss. Full restitution may take up to *a year or more* and some people never complete this stage.
— **Nursing responsibilities** include an assessment of where the patient is in the grief and mourning process, his efforts to resolve the loss, and the results. Intervention should focus on helping the patient move along the continuum of the three stages of loss and provide resources for discharge planning.

Specific Considerations, Potential Patient Outcomes, and Nursing Actions:

1) **Stage I:** **The patient will be able to use any non-destructive coping mechanisms to begin to deal with the loss;**
   Shock and
   Disbelief
   — accept any behavior that is not physically destructive; do not try to cut it off or limit it;
   — reinforce the occurrence of the loss while encouraging the pt. to talk about it; do not reinforce denial but rather, state, e.g., "It must be difficult to believe this is happening";
   — spend at least 15 mins. each shift talking and/or just sitting & listening to the pt.; allow the pt. to direct the conversation;
   — when appropriate, tell the pt. he is doing a good job of dealing with the loss;
   — flex visiting hours for family/friends to stay PRN; try to fulfill any pt. requests.

2) **Stage II:** **The patient will be able to verbally express an awareness of the loss and its impact on him:**
   Developing
   Awareness of
   the Loss
   — incorporate a discussion of the loss in your daily conversations with the pt. and/or family; appropriate questions might be: a) "How do you see the effect of what has happened to you?" b) "How has your family coped with what has occurred?"
   — when pt. begins to share sadness, encourage him to do so; sit & listen to what he says;
   — reiterate that what he is experiencing is normal for his situation;
   — involve the pt. in planning & doing some aspects of self care;
   — restate questions the pt. has asked so that he can explore the answers with your assistance;
   — make sure the pt. has ongoing situational supports to help him deal with the loss, e.g. friends, family, clergy.

3) **State III:** **The patient will be able to talk about the positive and negative aspects of the loss and make future goals:**
   Restitution
   — praise the pt.'s efforts to discuss the impact of the loss on his life; give positive reinforcement for future plans;
   — allow the pt. control over as much of his care & method of resolving the loss as possible.

Discharge Planning and Teaching Objectives/Outcomes

1) (Patient/Family/Significant Other) Can express sadness over the loss but also plan for the future.
2) Can verbalize how he copes with losses and what situational supports are most effective.

Recommended References

"Grief and Grieving" by George Engel. *American Journal of Nursing*, September 1965:93.
"Planning For Retirement" by Elizabeth E. May. *Health Values: Achieving High Level Wellness*, May-June 1977:133–136.
"Sharing a Tragedy" by Judith Breuer. *American Journal of Nursing*, May 1976:758–759.
"Solving the Riddle of Loss: 'Depression' and Other Responses." Filmstrips available from NURSECO, PO Box 145, Pacific Palisades, CA 90272.
"Traumatic Blindness: A Flexible Approach for Helping a Blind Adolescent." *Nursing '79*, January 1979:36–41.
"Therapeutic Touch: Searching for Evidence of Physiological Change" by Dolores Krieger, Erick Peper and Sonia Ancoli. *American Journal of Nursing*, April 1979:660–662.
"The Grieving Patient and Family" by Mary Jo B. Marks. *American Journal of Nursing*, September 1976:1488–1491.

© Margo Creighton Neal, 1980

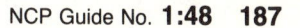

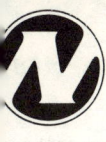

Steps in Writing a Nursing Care Plan

Definition: A nursing care plan is the tangible end result of the nursing process, and is a hallmark of professional nursing.

General Considerations:
— **Nursing process** is the scientific method of problem-solving applied to the functions of nursing. For nurses, it is a logical method of providing patient care based on five components or steps: (1) data collection; (2) nursing diagnosis; (3) goals/objectives/expected outcomes; (4) nursing actions; and (5) evaluation of patient response.
— **Initial nursing care plans** include the first four steps; following evaluation of the patient response, **on-going plans** include all components. Each step is outlined here and is accompanied by the corresponding standard of nursing practice as defined by the American Nurses' Association (ANA).

Step 1: DATA COLLECTION
ANA Standard: "The collection of data about the health status of the client/patient is systematic and continuous. The data are accessible, communicated and recorded."

1.1 **Conduct an admission interview** with the patient and/or family/significant other(s) as soon as possible (see NCPG #1:44, "Suggestions for Interviewing.").

1.2 **Acquire additional information** from observation, physical assessment, old chart, admitting sheet, doctor, or any source possible. **Consider the kinds of information** you need in order to **START** the care plan:
- physical, emotional, and psychological states?
- patient's perception of current illness and hospitalization?
- social, cultural, economic, religious, environmental influences?
- habits and activities of daily living?
- past experiences/history of illnesses?
- what other areas will you explore?

1.3 **Write out the data** on a nursing history/interview/assessment form (See NCPG #1:46, "Restoring +" form.). Use of such a form will provide you with a tool for systematic collection of the data, as well as making it available to other personnel.

1.4 Know that **initial data collection may be limited** by one or more variables, e.g. time, patient's condition. *Do the best you can at the time;* you will have later opportunities to gather additional data.

Step 2: NURSING DIAGNOSES:
ANA Standard: "Nursing diagnoses are derived from health status data."
2.1 Nursing diagnoses are the **end products of assessment;** they are those patient needs/problems/concerns that are the *independent* functions of nursing and require nursing interventions.
2.2 Making a nursing diagnosis is the process of **interpreting** the health status data for the purpose of defining a situation. This diagnositc process has three steps (Becknell & Smith, 1975):
   (1) *Extract* relevant facts and concepts from the data collected in Step 1;
   (2) *Sort and clarify* this information into groups that demonstrate relationships: What pieces of data go together? Are related? Is there a logical fit between some subjective and objective data?
   (3) *Interpret the data,* that is, *make a nursing diagnosis,* based on the groups or relationships you have identified.
2.3 Refer to NCPG #2:47 for the list of nursing diagnoses and the references at the end of this section.
2.4 Set **priorities** based on your nursing judgement; focus on these priority diagnoses rather than attempting to take care of all the needs/problems at once.

Step 3: GOALS/OBJECTIVES/EXPECTED OUTCOMES
ANA Standard: "The plan of nursing care includes goals derived from the nursing diagnoses."
3.1 Goals/objectives/expected outcomes (G/O/EOs) are both **long-term and short-term**.
3.2 Both are **behaviorally-stated in terms of what the patient will be doing,** not the nurse. The easiest way to do this is to use the stem, "The patient will . . ." This does not denote forcing; rather, it reflects a behaviorally-defined statement.
3.3 The **long-term G/O/EO is the desired end result of the illness or hospitalization.** Essentially, it will be a variation of *one* of the following:
   (1) For the patient with an *acute* illness who has no chronicity or disability:
       "The patient will return to his usual roles of (define these roles, e.g., work/family roles)."
   (2) For the patient with a *chronic* illness and/or some degree of disability:
       "The patient will adapt to and live within the limitations of (define the limitations and optimum level of functioning)."
   (3) For the *terminally ill* patient:
       "The patient will experience a peaceful and dignified death."
3.4 Each of the above long-term G/O/EOs must be **individualized to each patient**. A patient can have only one long-term G/O/EO at any given time, but it can change during hospitalization. You may not have sufficient data on admission to set a long-term G/O/EO; this may have to be done at a later date when more information is available.

3.5 **Short-term G/O/EOs are the desired end result of the nursing diagnoses.** The criteria for writing one includes that it be:
   (1) *Specific:* Use specific verbs to achieve this, e.g., "The patient will *talk* . . ." "The patient will *write* . . ."
   (2) *Measurable:* Include a standard of measurement, e.g., "The patient will talk about *feelings of loss of use of the arm.*" "The patient will write out a *24-hour menu for a 1500 calorie diet.*"
   (3) *Realistic:* Is the G/O/EO realistic for this patient? Is it possible for the patient to achieve it?
3.6 Specify a short-term G/O/EO for **every** nursing diagnosis you have made.

Step 4: NURSING ACTIONS

ANA Standard: "The plan of nursing care includes priorities and the prescribed nursing approaches or measures to achieve the goals derived from the nursing diagnosis."

4.1 Nursing actions reflect **how** you will intervene to help the patient reach the G/O/EOs. These actions are *specific to the short-term G/O/EO* and the corresponding nursing diagnosis. As each short-term G/O/EO is being met, the results feed into achievement of the long-term one.

4.2 Prescribe your nursing actions **clearly and concisely** so that other staff using the care plan will know what you expect them to do for the patient. Instead of writing "encourage," for example, spell out what you want staff to be doing when they are "encouraging."

4.3 Determine a period of time to implement these actions before evaluation is done, e.g., "Evaluate in 3 days." Write this on the care plan card.

Step 5: EVALUATION OF PATIENT RESPONSE

ANA Standard: "The client's/patient's progress or lack of progress toward goal achievement directs reassessment, reordering of priorities, new goal setting and revision of the plan of nursing care."

5.1 **Evaluate the patient's response to the nursing actions** in relation to the short-term G/O/EO. Has the latter been achieved?

5.2 **Has the identified need/problem been resolved?** If *yes*, then direct your focus to the next priority. If progress is being made but the G/O/EO has not been reached, you may wish to continue with all actions. If there is *no* progress, then determine the cause. It could be any of the following:
   (1) *The actions:* Are there other options you can try?
   (2) *The short-term G/O/EO:* Is it realistic for this patient? Does it need to be changed?
   (3) *The nursing diagnosis:* Is this the priority with the patient, or is there some other need/problem that is more pressing? Have new developments changed the priority?

5.3 **Revise** the care plan as necessary, according to your findings.

SUMMARY

Nursing care plans provide patients with organized, consistent care on a continuing basis. They reflect changes in the patient's health status.

Nursing process provides nurses with a professional model for providing nursing care. It is a dynamic, on-going process that reflects the independent functions of professional nursing.

Recommended References

How to Write Realistic, Workable Nursing Care Plans. A series of 4 sound filmstrips available from Nurseco, PO Box 145, Pacific Palisades, CA 90270.
"Nursing Diagnoses," *NCP Guide* #2:47, 2nd Ed., Nurseco, 1980.
Nursing Diagnosis and Intervention in Nursing Practice, by Claire Elaine Campbell. New York: John Wiley & Sons, 1978.
"Restoring +," *NCP Guide* #1:46, 2nd Ed., Nurseco, 1980.
Systems of Nursing Practice, by E. Becknell and D. Smith. Philadelphia: F.A. Davis Co., 1975.

© Margo Creighton Neal, 1980

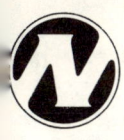

Teaching Patients: General Suggestions

GOAL: The patient/family/significant other will develop the necessary skills, self-confident attitude and knowledge for effective control of disease and disability and for solving problems of daily living within unavoidable or recommended limitations; the patient/family/significant other will prevent, through self-care and maintenance of health, recurrence of problem or avoidable complications.

General Considerations:

— Patient education programs & departments have increased in numbers and are presently available in most hospitals, of over 150 patients, throughout the U.S.

— Nurses who believe that **patient education is** an integral part of their **nursing** role and **responsibility** can seek to fulfill their patient's teaching needs through self continuing education and by compiling a resource list of ex-patients, persons with special language skills or sign language abilities, and nursing specialists on various disease entities who will serve as consultants and helpers. Many commercial teaching aids are now available to help with patient teaching.

— Remember, **timing and patient readiness are essential to effective learning.** If patient is in a process of grief and depression over a diagnosis or impact of surgery, or is overwhelmed with fear, s/he may not hear or absorb information. S/he may even refuse to listen or to believe anything you say . . . denying a need to learn. The patient should be permitted to progress and direct own learning at own pace, even if this means that some will not be ready for self-care at discharge. Preparation of a friend or family member is suggested; transfer to a convalescent hospital may be necessary. Referral to a community health nurse is often desirable.

— Refer to NCPG #1:31, "Responses to Loss: the Grief and Mourning Process," PRN. Plan consistent care of the patient with colleagues; reinforce reality; ask questions; take time to listen.

— Consider **a written or verbal contract,** identifying what specific changes in lifestyle and behavior are needed, desired and agreed to by patient, in order to maintain the desired level of health and disease control.

— **Use** or develop an **assessment form** to guide your interview of patient and family, to assist in developing a relevant, individualized teaching plan, and to serve as a permanent record along with patient/family education record of learning attained.

— Obtain a doctor's authorization to teach patient, if this is required by hospital policy.

— Refer to NCPG #1:50, "Teaching Patients: Specific Plan for Skills and Procedures."

Nursing Actions:
ASSESSMENT:
1) *Assess the patient/family's readiness to learn:*
   — emotional acceptance of condition, psychological adjustment, and willingness to talk about this in personal terms;
   — motivation and desire to learn, willingness and ability to modify life-style as indicated by disease/disability management or rehabilitation;
   — educational level of achievement; comprehension;
   — age and relevance of proposed teaching methods;
   — attention span; memory ability;
   — coordination (eye-hand, posture, balance, etc. as relevant);
   — vision (color and focus, acuity); hearing;
   — reading and writing ability;
   — ability to use telephone; to seek, accept and effectively use help;
   — ability to drive a car or use public transportation.

2) *Assess factors influencing teaching plan:*
   — patient's daily routine, employment conditions, family relationships, eating & sleeping patterns, travel, hobbies, use of time, responsibilities;
   — cultural and ethnic influences (dietary preferences), sexual or racial influences;
   — beliefs and attitudes re: health, illness, medical treatment;
   — is there a family member or friend who wants/needs to learn about patient's care? Can sessions be arranged to include this person, or be done at another time?
   — architectural constraints of home or living quarters, i.e. size or privacy of bathroom, number of steps, height of working surfaces, etc.

3) *Identify the important learning needs for a particular patient/family member/friend:*
   — disease pathology (cause, cure, control);
   — medication (purpose, untoward side effects, recommended dosage, administration);
   — diet (foods allowed, foods to be avoided, adaption for cultural preferences, menu selection when dining out, sample menus, food preparation);
   — activity (mental and physical rest, kind and amount of exercise, plans for leisure/recreation/sports, occupational adjustments);
   — personal health habits (smoking, drinking, coping with stress, special needs of skin, feet, hair, eyes, etc., use of assistive devices, prosthetics);
   — prevention of complications (signs and symptoms to be noted and reported, need for medical identification card);
   — community resources (address and phone number of community health agency, mutual self-help groups, vocational rehabilitation facilities, department of social services, etc.).

PLANNING:
1) Involve the family and friends (as well as the patient) in the planning, implementation and evaluation of the teaching program.
2) Establish specific, measurable, *realistic* objectives (expected outcomes); example: "Pt./S.O. can verbalize and/or demonstrate knowledge of. . . ." Arrange list of objectives in sequential steps, from simple to complex, considering also the patient's most pressing needs/problems/concerns.
3) Prepare an individualized, detailed lesson plan and assemble audio-visual teaching aids.
4) Consult sources of educational materials available for care of a given condition. Try to obtain both materials suitable for giving to patient and those recommended for teaching yourself.

IMPLEMENTATION:
1) Whenever possible, assign only one person to teach patient in order to minimize confusion, contradiction and incompleteness. Whenever possible, have that person be present when supplementary teaching is being done by a consultant specialist (dietician, volunteer ex-patient, pharmacist, etc.). Reinforce information as needed.
2) Schedule teaching sessions according to patient's receptivity (fatigue, distractibility, interest, readiness, comfort). Let patient set pace and choose topics of most interest.
3) Provide a quiet, well-ventilated, distraction-free setting for learning.
4) Provide information using visual aids; obtain feedback by asking questions; don't say, "Do you understand?" but rather, "Tell me how you can do this yourself," or, "How can you use this information in your care at home?" or, "Tell me what your situation is." This may help to reveal patient's feelings, perceptions, misconceptions and need for reiteration of facts. Correct gaps in knowledge or errors in thinking and repeat information PRN.
5) Remember that successful learning may come slowly; it takes many days of activity to regain losses of strength and endurance caused by immobility and delayed rehabilitation programs. It takes time to unlearn or relearn incorrect habits. Maintain optimism and patience. Compliment patient for effort and for each increment of learning.
6) Provide a means for patients to learn more (or reinforce what was taught). Consider supplying leaflets, written instructions, referrals to health and education service agencies, the name and number of a community health nurse or of an ex-patient successfully rehabilitated and willing to help. Attach a copy of the teaching record to the referral form.

EVALUATION:
1) Administer tests to patient to determine learning; use oral, written quizzes or return demonstrations.
2) Keep a written record of what has been **learned**, not just what was taught and by whom. Share this with nurse, family member or friend who will care for patient at home. Provide a means for the patient to evaluate his own learning and to sign record; save for use if patient is readmitted; then reactivate, update and review teaching plan.
3) Consider sending patient a letter following discharge to evaluate patient compliance and your teaching effectiveness.

Recommended References
"Forms That Facilitate Patient Teaching," by Rebecca Whitehouse. *American Journal of Nursing*, July 1979:1227–1229.
"Responses to Loss: the Grief and Mourning Process." *NCP Guide* #1:31, 2nd Ed., Nurseco, 1980.
"Teaching Patients: Specific Plan for Skills and Procedures," NCPG #1:50, 2nd Ed., Nurseco, 1980.
"What Does Your Patient Need to Know?" by Joan Kratzer. *Nursing 77*, December 1977:82–84.

© Margo Creighton Neal, 1980

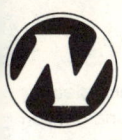

Teaching Patients: Specific Plan for Skills and Procedures

Goal: The patient will be able to (state the skill or procedure) by (set a completion date).

General Considerations:
— There are many skills and procedures that patients learn from nurses, e.g. testing urine for S&A, injecting insulin, suctioning and cleaning a tracheostomy tube.
— **Optimum results** can be expected when the nurse-teacher ensures the following:
   1) inclusion of basic learning conditions;
   2) teaching the skill or procedure in specific teaching steps; and
   3) allowing for individual differences in the patient-learner.
— **Basic Learning Conditions:** the three most important for teaching skills or procedures are:
   1:1 Contiguity: The individual steps of the procedure must be taught in continuous order or sequence. You may start with the first step and work to the last one, or start with the last step and work backwards; it doesn't matter as long as the steps are **in sequence**.
   1.2 Practice: This permits the patient to rehearse the sequence until each step is learned satisfactorily. Practice will be most effective when the patient distributes it over a period of time, e.g. several times a day for several days, rather than trying to perfect the entire sequence all at once.
   1.3 Feedback: This gives the patient knowledge of how s/he is doing. It is **the most important variable** in learning, and is highly motivating to the patient. Ask the patient to give you a return demonstration of what s/he has learned; critique it and correct any errors.
— **Specific Teaching Steps:** Organizing the content to be taught in the following order facilitates presentation and comprehension:
   2.1 Emotional Acceptance of condition: If patient is denying the condition or the need to learn the skill or procedure (denial is a common behavior), read NCP Guide #1:24.
   2.2 Assessment of learning needs: What does the patient **know now**? How can you build on this? What does s/he **need to know**?
   2.3 Explanation of Terminal Behavior: Tell the patient what s/he will be able to do when the learning is completed, e.g. test urine for S&A, inject insulin, etc.
   2.4 Demonstration of Procedure: Explain and demonstrate each step **in sequence**, repeating steps PRN.
   2.5 Return Demonstration by the patient: Give encouragement and feedback; make corrections PRN.
   2.6 Verbal Restatement of each step in the procedure by the patient, in **his own** words.
   2.7 Practice by the patient until mastery of the procedure is achieved.

— **Individual Differences:** Individuals learn, accept, and cope with things at different rates. Thus, the *time* a patient requires for each step, or the entire procedure, may vary widely. Some patients will require more practice, and more explanation, than others. Be patient, and caution your patient to be likewise.

The *learning/comprehension level* will vary from patient to patient, and you will need to adjust the level of your presentation accordingly. Ensure that you use terms, words, etc. that the patient understands.

Some patients may benefit from *reading* about the procedure. If possible, supply reading materials such as booklets, pamphlets, etc.

— In **summary**, then, include the three basic learning conditions in your teaching plan, follow the specific teaching steps as outlined in (2) above, and allow for individual differences.

Recommended References
"The Patient Manifesting Denial," *NCP Guide* #1:24, 2nd Ed., Nurseco, 1980.

© Margo Creighton Neal, 1980

NURSECO: independent nursing providers of continuing education

Dear Fellow Nurse:

Would you give us your evaluation of NCP Guides for Psychiatric and Mental Health Care? Your feedback can help us provide you with new and improved aids for continuing education. Just complete this card and drop it in the mail. Thank you very much.

Margo Neal, R.N., M.N.
Pat Cohen, R.N., M.A., Ed. M.
Phylis Cooper, R.N., M.N.
Joan Reighley, R.N., M.N.

What features of this Set are most helpful to you?

- goal
- general considerations
- problem areas
- objectives
- nursing actions
- discharge plans & teaching objectives
- references
- section on med-surg. conditions
- section on patient behaviors
- section on supplementary information
- others (please specify)

COMMENTS:

Suggestions for Additional NCP Guides

First Class
Permit No. 107
Pacific Palisades, Calif.

BUSINESS REPLY MAIL
No postage stamp necessary if mailed in the United States

Postage will be paid by

NURSECO
P.O. Box 145
Pacific Palisades, California 90272

"NOTES"

"NOTES"

"NOTES"

"NOTES"